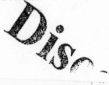

THE
SINGER'S
AND
ACTOR'S
THROAT

THE SINGER'S AND ACTOR'S THROAT

The Vocal Mechanism of the Professional Voice User and its Care in Health and Disease

NORMAN A. PUNT

FRCS ED, MRCS, LRCP, DLO

Laryngological Adviser to
The National Theatre
The English National Opera
and Laryngologist to
The Royal Shakespeare Company
The Royal Academy of Dramatic Art
The D'Oyly Carte Opera Company
The Birmingham School of Music

THIRD EDITION

William Heinemann
Medical Books Limited
London

FIRST PUBLISHED 1952
SECOND, REVISED, EDITION 1967
THIRD, REVISED, EDITION 1979

© Norman A. Punt 1979

ISBN 0 433 26451 9

Printed in Great Britain by
REDWOOD BURN LIMITED
Trowbridge & Esher

Preface to the Third Edition

This is a book mainly for singers and actors, but also for barristers, lecturers and public speakers, and for all whose profession entails considerable use of the voice. It is also intended for those concerned with the training of professional voice users, and thus are included teachers of singing and acting, speech therapists and elocutionists.

The aim has been to describe the mechanism of speech and song with correct emphasis on the importance of various details of structure and function so that the numerous factors concerned in beautiful singing and speaking may be understood and appreciated in proper perspective; and from the above to advise with regard to the *principles* on which *any* 'method' of speech or song should be based. In addition the book deals with matters affecting the care of the voice in health and during the course of those common and ubiquitous inflammations which, though no more than a nuisance to most of us, are minor catastrophes to professional voice users. The prevention and treatment of certain conditions due to wrong use or over-use of the vocal mechanism, and therefore particularly common in this group of people, are also discussed.

Unless the contrary is indicated the word 'singer' may be taken to refer also to other professional voice users—differences in action during other forms of phonation being indicated where necessary.

As Tickner Edwardes[76] pertinently remarks:

'A Doctor Dryasdust will manage to impart to the truths he meddles with a disastrous air of dullness and stagnation; but to walk in a fool's paradise of beautiful, artistic error is to lay oneself open to an infinitely worse fate. There never was a truth in Nature that was dull or uninteresting, except in its human presentment. There never was a pretty worthless fiction that did not show its dross and tinsel when brought out into the searching light of day.'

Experience has confirmed the opinion expressed by me 25 years ago that singers, actors and other professional voice users almost all go through a period some time in their careers when their voice gives them trouble and anxiety, and that they can be helped not only by specific treatment by the laryngologist, but also by a little understanding of structure and function and of what has gone wrong with the vocal mechanism. This applies both to students and to highly successful and experienced performers.

Many such artists and their teachers, who for professional reasons must all remain anonymous, have expressed appreciation of the former volume, and an ever-increasing number of enquiries has resulted in the publication of this new and revised edition.

Finally I would like to record my thanks to those who have helped directly or indirectly, in the production of the book; thus to my wife, my teachers, certain colleagues and patients, Mr. Oren Brown of the Juilliard School of New York, the library staffs of the Royal Society of Medicine, the Royal Institution and the Central Music Library, my publishers, and my secretary Mrs. Sue Gates.

Contents

1 Professional Voice Users:
  Their Mental Attitude and Peculiar Problems   1

2 Structure and Function of
  the Vocal Mechanism in Outline   14

3 Attributes Necessary for Fine Singing   33

4 Care and Use of the Voice in Health   48

5 Why Voices 'Break Down';
  Prevention and Treatment   61

6 Producers, Directors and Voices   82

7 Fallacies and Traditions   86

  BIBLIOGRAPHY   93

  INDEX   97

1
Professional Voice Users: Their Mental Attitude and Peculiar Problems

It has seemed best to begin this book by describing vocal problems in a general way with emphasis on the mentality common to perhaps 90 per cent. of singers and actors. All good teachers of medicine insist that one treats patients—individual men and women—not text-book examples of diseases and dysfunctions. Thus it would appear logical to give some account of the nature of singers and actors, that we may know at least with what manner of men and women we are dealing, before going on to the more impersonal description of structure, function and dysfunction. An additional reason for putting this chapter first is that of the many causes which lead to a person becoming a singer or actor, the stronger is frequently a psychological one. Complementary to this is the fact that, in spite of all scientific research, when the last graph has been studied, the final figures analysed and the ultimate equation resolved, a large factor amongst those determining the effect produced by a singer on his audience is also a psychological one. Although at first sight there may seem to be little point in describing the temperament commonly possessed by singers and actors in a chapter primarily intended for their perusal, we believe it to be important for reasons that will appear in due course.

No matter how diligently he studies or what attributes of voice, person or skill he may possess, it is one of the hard facts of the theatre that no performer is likely to gain lasting success unless he has a certain volatility—with an ability to sense the reactions of his audience as he conveys to them sentiments of situation and character. Actors and singers, therefore, are sensitive, excitable people—readily influenced, a prey to their emotions and reacting violently to changes in environment.

1

There are exceptions, but they are not common. I do not think anyone accustomed to working with theatre people would deny this. It has been called the artistic temperament and much nonsense and not a few jibes have originated from the phrase; yet it should not be difficult to understand, for if actors and singers were dull, phlegmatic, placid people, no one would go to the trouble of listening to them. So of course they may be excitable, neurotic, volatile, temperamental, changeable, moody, intemperate, vain, unstable and so on. But they are also usually pleasant, cheerful, grateful, generous personalities endowed with tremendous courage. Moreover they are not only artists, but artists whose medium is their own bodies, and the very nature of their Calling (Irving's word) with its uncertainties and rapidly changing emotional atmospheres, makes it no occupation for the lover of well-ordered placidity. Less the eternal amateur gets the wrong idea we must interpolate that the portrayer of emotion on the stage is *not* experiencing a like emotion at the time; but he would not so portray it if he were incapable temperamentally of sympathetically comprehending that emotion. As evidence one may cite the well-known difficulty in finding a satisfactory Juliet, no actress young enough to look the part having sufficient experience of life off the stage to be able to play it.

But this question of the psychology of actors has been dealt with by the great critic and essayist William Hazlitt in a fine-passage which is at once vindication and salutation:

'With respect to the extravagance of actors, as a traditional character, it is not to be wondered at. They live from hand to mouth, they plunge from want into luxury; they have no means of making money *breed* and all professions that do not live by turning money into money, or have not the certainty of accumulating it in the end by parsimony, spend it. Uncertain of the future they make sure of the present moment. This is not unwise. Chilled with poverty, steeped in contemp, they sometimes pass into the sunshine of fortune, and are lifted to the very pinnacle of public favour; yet even there they cannot calculate on the continuance of success, but are, "like the giddy sailor on the mast, ready with every blast to topple down into the fatal bowels of the deep!" Besides, if the young enthusiast, who is smitten with the stage, and with the public as a mistress, were naturally a close *hunks*, he would become or remain a city clerk, instead of turning player. Again, with respect to the habit of convivial indulgence, an actor, to be a good one, must have a great spirit of enjoyment in himself—strong impulses, strong passions, and a strong sense of pleasure: for it is his business to imitate the passions, and to communicate pleasure to others.'

That was written 150 years ago and it is still true, notwithstanding modern financial techniques arising out of taxation and accountancy.

Fame, wealth and realization of artistic ambition apart, the life of a leading International singer is not to be envied. These artists become unsettled by constant changes of scene and climate, by uncomfortable travelling from airport to airport and from hotel to hotel, and also by the lack of 'roots' with a home, family and close friends. Young singers, especially, suffer from insecurity and the disruption of personal attachments. It is not unusual for a consultation to start on the theme of 'laryngitis' and end with tears and the story of a broken engagement.

We must also remember (as Hazlitt wrote, in the idiom of his time) that although leading performers earn large incomes, they practice in an uncertain and overcrowded profession, are frequently forced to retire relatively young, and come into the financial category of casual labourers.

Special mention should be made of the agonizing art of the clown. The great drolls of the time—the 'comics' as they are now called—usually, in the writer's experience, endure agonies of anxiety and depression. Few professional people suffer as much as the player who must step upon a stage and make his audience laugh, knowing full well that if they don't laugh, he is not funny—and that no excuse or argument can mitigate a failure. The sad and worried clown is a heart-breaking sight, and the £2000 a week he may be earning is small consolation. If he ceases to be funny the money will stop—and very quickly too!

Any actor or singer will agree that all this is true, but some may wonder what it has to do with the throat and voice. It has a great deal to do with the vocal organ and its performance. The vocal mechanism may be healthy and undamaged, but the precision with which it responds to the subtle and intricate demands made upon it is so often affected by the state of mind and emotions of the performer, perhaps especially when it is concerned with the exceedingly delicate and complex series of co-ordinated movements which result in song. Tranquillity and confidence, anxiety set-aside, yet sensitivity to the emotions of the dramatic situation and of the participating audience, should be the player's aim. But this ideal is rarely achieved, and such failure is often a large factor in the singer or actor not making the most effective use of his voice. On occasions it may be the *only* cause of disaster, but in *any* dysfunction, or even disease, of the throat, this emotional factor may be of importance and this should never be forgotten, nor yet over-emphasized, by anyone concerned (the Management will usually blame the emotions, and the artist will probably rationalize according to personality; but the laryngologist has to evaluate all the possible stresses).

These disturbances take many forms. They are usual as 'first-night nerves'; all beginners suffer from them, as do most experienced artists, however fine; they are met with in an exaggerated form as the result of bad news or a fright, the victim being suddenly 'struck dumb' or speechless. Many long-standing speech defects have a similar aetiology.

So if the reader of these lines is a worried student thinking that he is exceptional in enduring such torments, he can at least be assured that they are not only frequent, but usual; most of his colleagues, his seniors and the famous leaders of his profession, suffer similarly, although they often use their acting ability to disguise them off the stage as well as on.

Before a First Night, I once visited a dear friend with sixty years experience of the Stage and with many fine performances behind her—and a 'simple' part to play—to find her trembling with fright and saying 'O, why do I do it?'. (Her performance was most moving and immaculate, and the un-knowing must have thought it so easy.)

Professional confidences must be inviolate, but one may quote from published writings of great artists of the past:

First, Caruso[74]: 'Of course I am nervous. Each time I sing I feel there is someone waiting to destroy me, and I must fight like a bull to hold my own. The artist who boasts he is never nervous is not an artist—he is a liar or a fool.'

Next Irving—not an actor one associates with nervousness—yet Ellen Terry[79] writing of his early days at the Lyceum when his first-night playing of Hamlet had been below his achievements on tour, and he had 'seemed stiff from self-consciousness,' blamed his habit of waiting for his cue in the wings: 'I begged him to give up that dreadful paralysing waiting at the side for his cue.'

Again, of Frederick Robson, we read: 'He was very nervous, and his sufferings on a First Night were painful to behold. He took too little rest, and was too much the slave of excitement' (F. Whyte[80]).

Finally the temperamental qualities necessary for a fine singer—an 'artist' rather than a 'voice machine'—are summed up by Tetrazzini[54] as 'imagination, feeling, sympathy, insight, magnetism and personality,' without which, however good they may be technically, they leave audiences cold, for they are cold themselves.

We have now outlined the form and effects of the almost universal anxiety or 'nervousness' which, at some time or another in some degree, attacks nearly all singers and actors by reason of their Calling and the mental make-up usually required for its practice—a perfectly understandable phenomenon resulting from having to face an audience uncertain of their reception and of the critics, managers and others on whom the player's reputation and livelihood depend.

But there is a special anxiety, suffered as far as our own observation goes by all singers and many actors at some period of their career, associated with the health of the vocal mechanism itself. The singer, particularly, knows that his professional reputation, income and frequently the greater part of the enjoyment derived from his very life depend on the health of his respiratory tract; and the site where inflammation or injury commonly produces most impairment of vocal quality, temporarily or permanently, is in the larynx itself. He therefore fears for the health of his larynx, thinking that too many missed shows on account of laryngeal trouble may injure his reputation for reliability, or even that serious permanent damage will for ever ruin his voice and career.

The larynx to the singer is what hands are to the surgeon, limbs to the dancer or eyes to the marksman. But, unlike the latter, the singer's throat is subject to a multitude of strange sensations which he usually tries to analyse, often with the handicap of very erroneous ideas of structure, function and what he calls 'voice production'. Almost assuredly he becomes obsessed with such notions, which serve only to increase his anxiety and may lead to injurious habits or treatments.

Obviously, if a professional voice user fears he may have some disease or injury of his throat he cannot do better than consult a laryngologist who can, at least, examine the larynx and readily detect the presence or absence of serious damage; and, if he is accustomed to the particular problems of these patients, can assess fine degrees of imperfection of function. Frequently the result of such examination is reassuring, and few things do so much to restore the morale of a singer as the re-assurance coupled with the sharing of responsibility that a consultation brings about. Should, however, the patient's fears be realized, advice and treatment can be prescribed.

The above is perhaps more applicable to long-standing troubles of the vocal mechanism. Another very common type of problem is that of the singer who develops a sudden attack of throat inflammation during the course of an engagement, or perhaps just before an especially important performance or audition. He does not want to miss performances unless absolutely essential; his reputation for reliability is a precious asset, financial loss to him and his management may be considerable, and he hates to break faith with his public. The theatre tradition that 'the show must go on' is a noble one. In fact if a player is well enough to be up and about, almost the only excuse for non-appearance *is* vocal dysfunction. Neither, however, does he want to give a performance far below his best; and, most important of all, he must not appear if his throat is in such a condition that singing or acting involves the risk of long-standing or permanent damage. The way to approach this common problem of 'to sing or not to sing' is to regard it as a duty incumbent upon the patient and the laryngologist *to do everything possible to 'get him through,'* **short of** *risking serious damage to the vocal mechanism.* Again sharing responsibility is a help to the singer physically and mentally.

In discussions about vocal dysfunction caused by over-use of the voice or by upper respiratory inflammation, the opinion is often expressed that there is no point in treatment and that all that is required is for the player to take a week or two's rest from the theatre. Could any advice be more psychologically inadequate when given to a performer whose livelihood depends so much on the health of the throat and who is perfectly understandably worried about it? In practice it is about as helpful as advising a busy doctor or the mother of a young family to take a week's holiday every time he or she catches a 'cold'! For an artist to miss a performance is a serious thing, and the fortunes of a play or opera, involving perhaps thousands of pounds, the player's reputation and many people's living for months to come may depend on getting a laryngeal condition well in a few days rather than weeks.

While on this point it is as well to say a word about the professional doctor-patient relationship between singer and laryngologist. It is one of the fundamental principles of ethical medical practice in this country that nothing learnt by a doctor in consultation with a patient may be disclosed to a third party without the patient's approval. No member of a theatrical company will fail to realize the importance of this in his own particular case. But circumstances do arise where it is to everyone's advantage to discuss a singer's immediate future with the latter's manager, agent or producer; and, with the singer's approval, such a three-cornered consultation can often do much to clear up a situation which has been embarrassing and nerve-racking to all concerned, and possibly threatened the fortunes of a production and the course of a singer's career.

Yet another psychological factor which may have a direct bearing on the health of the vocal mechanism must now be mentioned. Most singers and actors are friendly, talkative, sociable people, and consequently their leisure hours are often spent in conversation, frequently in a noisy gathering, when the larynx should be resting to compensate for the additional strain thrown upon it during performance. In addition the consumption of alcohol and tobacco, and the breathing of vitiated atmospheres, if indulged in to excess, is damaging to the mucous membrane covering the throat and to the vocal cords themselves. The direct cause of the damage is mechanical, but the underlying cause lies in the psychological make-up of the player, and as this is the more important consideration both for prevention and treatment it is appropriately mentioned here.

The restless, rushing-about type of locomotion to which stage people frequently become habituated also tends towards impairment of co-ordinated control of muscular action, including muscles involved in breathing and singing.

Another variety of upset which may, by reason of its psychological effect, act adversely is the emotional stress often occasioned by personal relationships. We have always believed in the definition that distinguishes between professional and amateur by stating that whereas the former can do his job when he doesn't feel like it, the latter can't when he does; but nevertheless it takes a quite exceptional artist to endure emotional unrest, week in and week out, without his or her work suffering in the long run. That singers and actors are peculiarly liable to such upsets is well known; if they were not so it is unlikely they would be able to convey emotion to an audience, as has already been explained. Some Managements are more sympathetic than others!

So far this chapter has been concerned with the psychology of singers and actors, its bearing on vocal function and the peculiar problems which arise from any suspicion that all is not well with the health of these organs. It contains many generalizations, but we believe any actor or singer will admit that the picture is, generally speaking, a true one, and will probably recognize certain characteristics in himself.

Apart from the obvious though frequently neglected desirability of including in such a work as this a general description of the nature and way of life of actors and singers, the value of the foregoing to the actor or singer reading this book in search of helpful advice lies in the importance of understanding and allowing for these psychological factors in the diagnosis, treatment and general management of any vocal dysfunction in himself. Such understanding is important to the patient as well as to his doctor, for no treatment is likely to succeed without the willing and intelligent co-operation of the patient. The rôle of the doctor as the 'mystery man' of medicine is, in more enlightened circles, showing signs of changing. The wise doctor today takes his patient into his confidence to a degree determined in each individual case by the judgment of the patient's mentality, understanding and intelligence.

Though the above factors are important in *any* throat condition affecting a singer or actor, their importance naturally varies in proportion to the degree in which any individual's vocal trouble is due to nervous causes rather than to disease or injury. And in so far as a condition has a psychological basis, the treatment must be by psychological methods—though, lest the words convey to the reader some false conception exploited by recent novels and films, these seldom involve more than a frank and friendly discussion between patient and doctor of the former's difficulties, worries and problems. This discussion, in itself, the patient doing most of the talking, is usually helpful by reason of the mental relief occasioned by the latter sharing the responsibility which has been weighing on him with his doctor, in whom, as the consultation proceeds, he should gain confidence. The doctor's part in this discussion usually consists of no more than simple explanation and, where possible, reassurance. This explanation is of great value and when, after examining the throat, reassurance can be added, the greater part of the singer's worries—and hence his difficulties—are often found to have vanished and he leaves the consulting room 'singing with joy and relief'. Explanation must, of course, be appropriate to each individual person, but as far as the psychological factors influencing singing are concerned the foregoing pages should suffice.

As has been said, anxiety can usually be relieved by *discussion, the sharing of responsibility, explanation and reassurance.* There are occasions, however, where the use of sedative or stimulant drugs, for a short time and after very careful consideration, is justified. The important point is that they should be discontinued as soon as possible, or their use reserved for exceptional circumstances; they should be prescribed by the *doctor,* and only *after* discussion and consideration. On no account should the singer be tempted by the pernicious lure of patent medicine advertisements or by the well-meant advice of friends to try this, that or the other 'tonic,' 'nerve medicine' or sleeping tablet. Without the procedure previously described, such drugs are very unlikely to be of use, may well do harm and may become a dangerous habit, making the eventual treatment of the singer's problem much more difficult to deal with.

Recently there has been some interesting discussion about a type of medicament known as a 'beta-blocker' (originally introduced for certain cardiac conditions). These substances, taken by mouth about half-an-hour before performance, do have the function of slowing the heart-rate and 'quietening the palpitations' of nervous performers. Like any other artificial aid they should be reserved for special occasions, such as First-Nights and important auditions, but the author can confirm the original reports by Dr. Ian James[61] and others (which recorded their action in instrumentalists undergoing the ordeal of examination by a panel of judges). Phillipson,[65] and Critchley and Henson[57], may also be consulted.

It is relevant here to consider the question of *alcohol*, although most performers (contrary to sensational journalism) are abstemious. Taken in moderation for enjoyment or good-fellowship—and preferably *after* performance—wines and beers, or a measure of spirits, do no harm. But alcohol taken before performance in an attempt to 'quieten the nerves' or 'settle the emotions' defeats these objectives, very soon leads to excess, and thence to disaster and the fatal, 'polite', label of 'unreliable'—by which time the 'nerves' are worse than ever. In addition, strong spirits—enough to warm-up the skin on a cold winter's day—will also cause engorgement of the blood-vessels of a performer's throat and vocal cords, with resultant coarsening of his vocal tone. The end result is the pathetic example of an—often brilliant—performer, with a weak 'gin-and-midnight' voice, unsure of his lines or movements and, in a very strictly disciplined profession, unemployable.

For completeness, 'drugs', in the newspaper sense of the term, must be mentioned. Habituation does not take long and inevitably leads to disaster. The smoking of cannabis irritates the larynx and the damage may be permanent. The lower members of the 'pop singer' fraternity may think they are merely following the fashion and copying some millionaire 'star'. They must be told that along with 99 per cent of their colleagues such ambitions are highly unlikely to be fulfilled—and the more and 'harder' the drugs they take, the more surely are they heading for failure.

Wherever the solution to the problem of anxiety may lie, it certainly cannot be solved by alcohol or drugs. We have tried to indicate the general line of treatment, but will add the suggestion of diverting the patient's thoughts, for part of the day at least, into other channels. James Agate[72] put the matter so happily, unerringly selecting the two most appropriate authors of English classic literature, that we cannot do better than quote this passage from his autobiography: '. . . Johnson tells Boswell that to attempt to think down distressing thoughts is madness. A man so afflicted must divert such thoughts and not combat with them. Boswell asking whether a course of chemistry would be helpful, Johnson said chemistry, or ropedancing, or anything that would provide a retreat for the mind. Mrs. Crupps's remedy ran on similar lines: "You are a young gentleman, Mr. Copperfull, and my adwice to you is, to cheer up, Sir, to keep a good heart, and to know your own walue. If you was to take to skittles, now, which is healthy, you might find it divert your mind".' Our one qualification would be to insist that the diversion should not involve any activity likely to add further strain to the body generally or the larynx itself.

Of comparable importance to the effect of anxiety on co-ordinated muscular action is the frequently neglected effect on the *lubrication* of various moving parts of the throat. This also will be more fully described later, but it is as well to state here that the mouth and tongue are lubricated mainly by saliva, and the pharynx and larynx mainly by mucus. The few large glands which secrete (pour out) the saliva and the very many minute glands which secrete mucus are influenced in their function partly by psychological factors. Anxiety causes a reduction in their output, and consequently produces the most troublesome dry mouth and throat with tongue clinging to the roof of the mouth—experienced and dreaded by all public performers, though strangely neglected by medical men.

In recent years the present writer has become more and more impressed with the importance of this lubrication. It is remarkable how much punishment a well-lubricated larynx will stand, whilst a dry throat is a constant trial to the performer. If the dryness persists even when anxiety has been largely alleviated, one may try to stimulate the mucous and salivary glands, so that they produce an adequate quantity of thin secretion, by sucking a lemon-drop or lozenge, by using a harmless spray to wash away sticky, inspissated mucus, by a certain iodine-containing preparation, or in severe cases by giving a drug which actively stimulates the secretory nerve-supply to the glands themselves.

Though generally applicable to most professional voice users, this chapter so far has considered mainly actors and singers. We will conclude by discussing problems peculiar to the other groups who habitually make much use of their voices in the practice of their professions or trades.

The **clergy** have given their name to a condition known as 'clergyman's sore throat'. Though by no means confined to that Order, the manner of declamation employed during a service may be one of its causes. But it is pleasing to note that in the quarter-century which has elapsed since the preparation of the first edition of this book what was described as 'the ubiquitous clergyman's drone or wail' has become much rarer, so perhaps suggestions that some better method of declamation should be taught to divinity students have been adopted. Similar attention seems happily to have been given to church singing, although one still sees choristers who have suffered vocal damage from injudicious endeavours.

Cantors of synagogues present with a problem all their own, which will not be discussed in detail.

Academic lecturers and **school-teachers** would appear to be divided into those who make an effort to speak clearly and effectively and those who make no effort at all. Nervousness and the traditional Englishman's fear of making himself conspicuous may account for some of the latter group. The suffering and waste of time endured by students whose teachers will not take the trouble to learn how to speak to a class is appalling. We remember some of the scores of lecturers we have listened to in the past and recall a few whose style and delivery were masterly, some who were adequate and some who should never have been permitted to address a class (the latter group sadly including some fine intellects, many of whose *writings* were models of clarity and exposition). The only solution to this problem is for academic bodies to refuse to appoint to teaching positions any whose lecturing abilities have not been tested and found satisfactory.

Barristers must be considered vocally as having to combine the special skills of lecturer and actor. Their success depends partly on presenting their cases with clarity and logic, and partly on arousing sympathy by histrionic methods. Some would deny the latter contention, but in certain types of trial, even today, it can hardly be doubted.

On the subject of **politicians** one might be sarcastic, but judging from broadcasts it must be admitted that the *manner* of their delivery is improving. We shall therefore be content with merely mentioning the obvious importance of the subject to all political speakers.

Lastly is included a numerous class of **salesmen** of various articles and commodities, but especially those whose task it is to effect sales largely by argument and persuasion; this covers an enormous field, and a little reflection will lead to realization of the diversity of men whose business efficiency is seriously reduced by vocal dysfunction, and in whom the proper use and care of the voice is of first importance. Particularly in this class should be mentioned the friendly, often hail-fellow-well-met, type of business man who sells his goods or signs his contracts over a drink and a smoke or a West End dinner table. His problems vocally are not dissimilar to those of the friendly and talkative actor.

2
Structure and Function of the Vocal Mechanism in Outline

This chapter is intended to tell the professional voice user all he needs to know about the structure and function of the vocal mechanism in health, and no more. It is purposely dogmatic, and has been made as simple as possible.

'It is certainly, at first glance, a matter for wonder that men could pass their whole lives in the pursuit of the craft, and yet manage to preserve uncorrupted a faith which seems so readily, and at so many points, assailable. But it must be remembered that any observation of the inner life . . . was then an extremely difficult thing' (Tickner Edwardes[76]).

There is no point in the singer filling his head with too great a knowledge of the anatomy and physiology of the organs concerned with singing. Such details, though commonly included in works intended only for the singer, are of no more use to him than a description of the shoulder joint would be to a cricketer, or the visual apparatus to a marksman. This is supported by the statement of Sir Arthur Keith[22] that when learning to play golf he found his great anatomical knowledge no use to him—though he stressed that it might have been valuable to a teacher. Nor are singers likely to be equipped with the scientific grounding necessary for the understanding of such complexities. As has been truly stated by others, the various individual parts of the vocal mechanism cannot be separately controlled by the singer—not even to the extent that a violinist or pianist can control his wrists and finger joints—and any attempt to exert such conscious control is undesirable and ineffective. Melba[78]—one of the few singers who possessed some accurate knowledge of vocal health and action—wrote that we have no conscious control over these structures, and that if marked sensations are noticed in the throat muscles when singing there must be some unnecessary tension which will injure the voice. We even find ourselves to a considerable degree in sympathy with H. Plunket Greene[45] when he advises the beginner to avoid the 'anatomical jargon man,' stating that a knowledge of anatomy is useless to the singer and will only 'worry him into senseless solicitude about organs whose movements are mainly automatic'.

However, we have observed that all singers eventually acquire some theory of vocal function in singing—in fact the first few minutes of a consultation are frequently taken up by listening whilst the singer expounds his own views. Nearly every one of them has a theory differing in some regard from the others; and the various ideas have been compounded partly from fallacious or ill-understood teaching or books, and partly from the sensations experienced in the throat whilst singing. They are therefore erroneous in one or more important points. This, in itself, might not matter, but unfortunately singers tend to indulge in certain injurious methods of singing based on such false conceptions; then, when vocal troubles begin to bother them, they go back each to his own pet theory of function and try to diagnose the cause of their difficulties in accordance with these theories, and to administer suitable treatment, which usually makes matters worse. It would seem, therefore, that singers feel the need for some knowledge of structure and function, and this chapter will consequently be devoted to a simplified account based on scientific evidence and observation, avoiding as far as possible both discussion of points still to be elucidated and the closing of such gaps with insufficiently tested theory or conjecture.

The vocal mechanism is a **reed** instrument. The vibratile parts of the larynx known as vocal cords are *not* cords or strings, but really folds or ledges having only one free border, so comparisons with stringed instruments are invalid. It might be compared to an organ having only one pipe and a double reed, but the reed and the pipe, being made of contractile living tissue, can be varied in consistency, shape and dimensions; consequently a large range of notes with count-less variations and rapid changes in pitch, intensity and timbre (quality) can be produced. Thus the mechanism consists of:

1. **Lungs**—representing *bellows* and supplying a stream of air which passes up the trachea (windpipe) to impinge on the

2. **Vocal Cords**—causing them to vibrate in the manner of a *double reed*, thus throwing the air-stream into a series of complex vibrations. This vibrating column of air now passes through the

3. **Pharynx (Throat) and Mouth**—which act as *a series of resonators* and selectively amplify to varying degrees of intensity its fundamental tones and various overtones (harmonics).

Vowel sounds are produced when the air-stream is continuous; *consonants* by more or less complete interruptions of the stream by interposition in various ways of tongue, teeth, lips, etc. Sing-ing, for the most part consisting of long phrases, emphasizes vowels. Speech, particularly conversation rather than decla-mation, emphasizes consonants. The contrast is especially marked if, for example, English and German are considered rather than Italian and French—which is one of the reasons why the latter are easier to sing.

Essential details illustrated by simple line diagrams (Figs. 1, 2 and 3) will now be given of the points just mentioned.

1. **The Lungs** are constructed of tissue which is elastic, and are contained within the closed cavity of the chest. If this cavity were to be punctured, the lungs' elasticity would cause them to collapse and expel their contained air. With an intact chest wall, however, the lungs are subjected to a pressure which is *less* than that of the atmosphere, so that they are always somewhat expanded. Now if the ribs are raised in front and the dome-shaped sheet of muscle (the diaphragm) separating the chest from the abdominal cavity descends, the size of the chest cavity will be increased, the pressure within it will tend to fall further, and the lungs will be sucked outwards (expand), and air will be drawn into their contained tubes and cavities via the windpipe

(trachea). This is *inspiration*.

If now the ribs descend and the diaphragm rises, the lungs will contract and air will be expelled in expiration, thus providing the stream of air passing up the windpipe which is necessary for speech or song.

A trained speaker or singer controls *inspiration* by disciplined co-ordination of muscles of chest, abdominal wall and diaphragm. During vocalisation, *expiration* is controlled by the first two groups of muscles, the ascending diaphragm being in relaxation. The phrase 'diaphragmatic breathing' is often misused: it may be employed when discussing inspiration, but during expiration many singers refer to the diaphragm when the active muscles concerned are really those of the abdominal wall. (For a fuller account see Wyke).[33, 34]

2. **The Larynx** is a complicated organ consisting of a cartilaginous framework containing a system of muscles and joints. Its main function is that of a valve to protect the lungs from foreign-bodies, but we shall only consider its function in speech and song.

The important *vibratile* part of the larynx consists of the pair of *vocal cords*. These are situated at the top of the trachea (windpipe) and project like shelves or ledges from the side of the larynx into the air stream (see Figs. 1, 2 and 3). Their front ends are close together; but at their rear ends are a pair of joints controlled by muscles acting in such a way that these ends can be brought together or moved apart. The space between the cords is therefore roughly triangular, with its apex at the front (see Fig. 3). This space, through which all air entering or leaving the trachea (windpipe) must pass, is known as the *glottis*.

During inspiration the glottis is wide. During expiration (without phonation) the glottis is narrower. And during expiration accompanied by speech or song the free borders of the vocal cords are brought almost parallel and in contact, as the tracheal air-stream passes through the narrow glottic slit the edges of the vocal cords are thrown into rapid vibration, both vertically and horizontally. The air-stream is thus converted into a rapid series of puffs which consequently form a tone. The *rate* of these vibrations largely determines the fundamental *pitch* of the note produced at the larynx (e.g. 256 double vibrations per second for middle C). But the cords do not merely vibrate as a whole; they also vibrate in segments, and these *segmental vibrations* add *harmonics (overtones)* to the fundamental cord tone.

It is as well to emphasize again that *the so-called vocal cords are not strings, but reeds* of variable shape, dimensions and stiffness. A good analogy was made by Paget[46] when he compared them to the lips of a bugler.

3. **The Resonating Cavities of Pharynx (Throat) and Mouth.**

If a tuning-fork is struck and held in air it emits a comparatively weak note; but if its foot is then held against a suitable hollow structure (such as a cigar-box with a hole in it) the note sounds very much louder. Similarly the intensity of the sound produced by the vibrating part of a musical instrument such as the reed of an organ (or a string of a violin) is weak; but by the construction of the instrument this intensity becomes very much increased—by the organ-pipe and its contained air (or the hollow body of the violin). This phenomenon is known as *resonance*. The augmenting effect of a resonator on a tone is greater the nearer the pitch of the tone corresponds to the natural pitch of the resonator; and in simple cases such effects are fairly easily predictable—such as in the organ, where there exists a separate reed, each with its own pipe, for each note. But in the case of the human voice, the cord tones, as has been shown, consist of fundamental tones and a complex series of harmonic partials (overtones), and there are at least two very important resonators, one communicating with the other, by which the cord tones are modified. And moreover, by reason of the muscular components in their walls (see Fig. 1) these cavities can be varied in shape, dimensions, consistency of their walls and size of openings. When one considers the number of variables in the composition of the cord tones, and in the resonating cavities v.hich modify these various components, one no longer wonders at the enormous range of vocal expression of the human voice, the ease with which a previously heard voice can be distinguished from others—nor at the fact that singing can never be other than a chancy business, no one being able to predict with any certainty the potentialities of a completely untrained, unused singing voice (see Chapter 3 for fuller discussion of the latter problem).

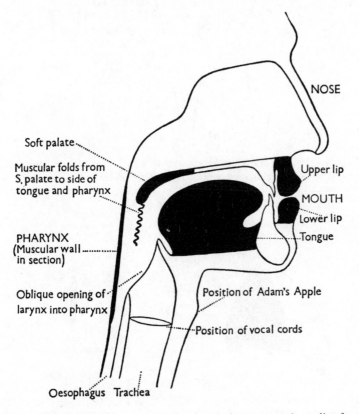

FIG. 1.   The resonating cavities of mouth and pharynx seen in outline from the side.

Muscular structures whose mobility varies the shape and dimensions (and therefore effect) of these resonators are shown in black.

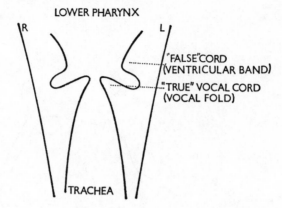

FIG. 2.   Diagram of a vertical cross section of the larynx in the frontal plane; after Chevalier Jackson, who states that 'the so-called vocal cords are not much like either cords or bands; they are really folds, pyramidal in cross section; the edge is not thin and sharp'.

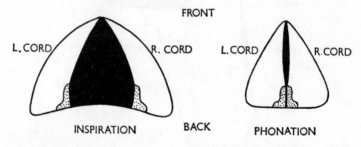

FIG. 3.   Diagrammatic representation of vocal cords ('Folds') in outline from above. Note that each cord has only one free edge—the inner one.
   The glottis is shown in black.
   The stippled structures represent a pair of articulated cartilages, partly inbedded in the cords, whose pivotal and sliding actions (controlled by several muscles) widen and narrow the glottis, by parting or opposing the cordal edges. (Only an approximate representation is possible in two dimensions.)

In brief, the human **pharynx** consists of an irregularly shaped tube leading from the larynx below to the back of the nose above. It communicates in front for part of its length with another resonating cavity, the **mouth.** As has been shown (see

Fig. 1) these cavities can be varied by action of the muscular components of their walls—also by movements of the lower jaw and by raising, lowering or tilting the larynx as a whole.

In addition there are other cavities whose resonating effect has been discussed inconclusively many times and at great length. In the present state of our knowledge it would probably be fair to say that the **chest cavity** may add volume and 'richness', especially in lower ranges of the voice; and that the resonating effect of the **nasal sinuses** (hollow spaces in the skull communicating with the nose) and **nasal cavities** is likely to be slight. There is little doubt that the pharynx, and to a lesser extent the mouth, are the most important resonating cavities.

In addition to the above simplified account of structure and function, it is necessary to say something of the lining of the respiratory tract. In general, the inside of the mouth and most of the pharynx is covered with a tough membrane, as, mercifully, are the vocal cords. The nose, upper pharynx and most of the larynx *except* the vocal cords are covered with a more delicate membrane. Situated in these lining membranes, but especially in the nose and in the larynx just above the vocal cords (but not in the cords themselves), are innumerable minute glands which secrete ('pour out') thin mucus. This mucus acts as a lubricant—it is the 'oil' in which the moving parts of the pharynx and larynx, especially the cords, function. The mouth, however, is lubricated mainly by saliva, secreted by a few large glands whose ducts open beneath the tongue and inside the cheek.

Another factor in this lubricating mechanism is the cleansing action brought about by innumerable microscopical cilia (tiny hairs or lashes) situated in these membranes. The cilia keep up a constant beating or waving motion and thus cause a continuous sheet of mucus to move from front to back of nose and down the pharynx, where it is swallowed. The nasal sinuses (hollow spaces in the skull communicating with the nose) are also lined with ciliated mucous membrane. So also are the trachea and bronchial tubes, their cilia moving the mucous sheet upwards towards the larynx. Thus the respiratory tract is kept lubricated and free from dust, and the inspired air is moistened and warmed.

Whenever the singer or actor happens to think about the structure and function of his vocal mechanism he is advised to keep clear in his mind this, deliberately simplified, conception of bellows, vibrator and resonators. This account can be elaborated for those who are interested, but every performer should at least understand the fundamental nature of the instrument.

Many singers need read no more of this chapter, but teachers, and those of their pupils who wish to know something of acoustics, and how variations in the actions of the structures concerned might affect the tone produced, may continue. The subject is complex and most research produces inconclusive or contradictory results, largely because so many frequently varying factors are concerned, that while one or two changes are being studied, some alteration in another part of the mechanism is neglected. It is not possible to measure all the many variables at the same time, so the following account of how changes in the vocal structures might, on physical grounds, affect the tone produced must be largely theoretical.

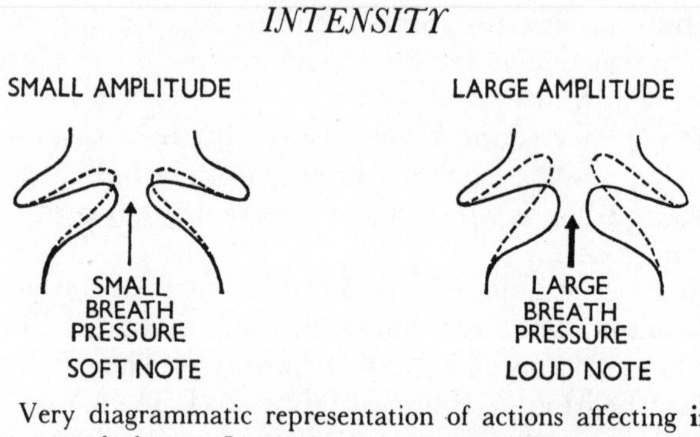

INTENSITY

SMALL AMPLITUDE   LARGE AMPLITUDE

SMALL BREATH PRESSURE   LARGE BREATH PRESSURE

SOFT NOTE   LOUD NOTE

FIG. 4.   Very diagrammatic representation of actions affecting **intensity** of a note at the larynx. Increasing breath pressure increases amplitude of cord vibrations and thus increases intensity of the note.

However, the vibrations are not simply vertical but include a complex rolling, lateral component. There are also changes in the exact portion of the cordal edges coming into opposition, and in the duration of opening, closing and shut phases of the cycle.

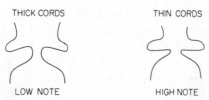

FIG. 5(*a*). Thinning of the cordal edges during singing raises the pitch of the note.

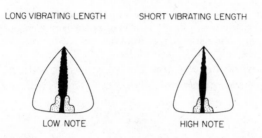

FIG. 5(*b*). Shortening the vibrating lengths of the cords is one way of raising pitch—e.g. falsetto mechanism, and flute voice.

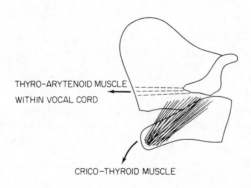

FIG. 5(*c*). More usually pitch is raised by contraction of the crico-thyroid muscle rocking the cricoid and arytenoid back on the thyroid, thus lengthening, but also stretching the cord, and so increasing its elasticity and tension.

PITCH (II)

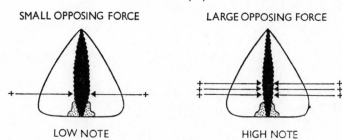

Fig. 6.   Increasing adductor force opposing cords, and raising breath-pressure, will raise pitch. (N.B. This manoeuvre may cause a singer to sing sharp, and also damage cordal surfaces and tire muscles—see text.)

The duration of the opening, closing and shut *phases* of the vocal cord movements may also vary with pitch changes.

PITCH (III)

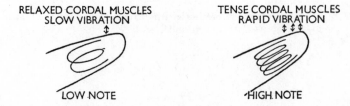

Fig. 7(*a*).   Theoretically, increasing the firmness or tension of the muscle fibres within the cords, makes them 'springier' and thus raises pitch—although these actions are disputed.

   (N.B. Excessive use of muscle tension causes tiredness—'myasthenia' —see text.)

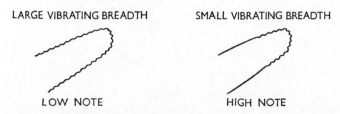

Fig. 7(*b*).   The smaller the *mass* of the portion of the cord actually vibrating, the higher the pitch.

A **tone** has three attributes, known as **intensity, fundamental pitch** and **quality (timbre).** The first two of these can be referred to precisely, but the third can only be described in terms of the sensations experienced by the listener, though the components responsible for it can be analysed. Thus, when a given note is sung (or sounded):

its *intensity* determines how *loud* we hear it,

its *fundamental pitch* determines its *position in the musical scale,*

its *quality (timbre)* determines whether it affects us as being *'rich,' 'bright,' 'clear,' 'fluty,' 'dark,' 'lyrical,' 'dramatic,' 'tender,' 'thin,' 'shrill,'etc., etc.*

Now imagine a column of air moving up the windpipe being thrown into vibration between the vocal cords, and these vibrations being further modified by the resonators, to form complex air-waves emerging from the mouth resulting in a tone. Some of the factors which are responsible for the characteristics of that tone are probably as follows:

1. INTENSITY depends on
    (a) *amplitude of cord vibrations* which depends on *breath pressure;*
    (b) accuracy with which the *resonators are tuned to the fundamental pitch.*

2. PITCH depends on *frequency of cord vibrations* which mainly depend on
    (a) *length, thickness, breadth and stiffness of the vibrating parts of the cords;*
    (b) *muscle force tending to close the glottis (oppose the cords);*
    (c) *breath pressure;*
    (d) *time relationships of opening, closing and shut phases of vocal cord movements.*

3. QUALITY (TIMBRE) depends on *harmonic partials (overtones)* which depend on
    (a) *segmental vibration of the cords* (manner uncertain);
    (b) *selective amplification of certain of these overtones by particular shape, dimensions and consistency of walls of the series of resonators (especially pharynx and mouth).*

In addition the particular *vowel sound* on which the note is sung *depends on resonator action*—and particularly on the augmentation of two or three particular partials.

It will be realized that the physiology and physics of song and speech are complex! Nor will it occasion surprise that the relative importance of all these theoretically possible actions is still (and probably always will be) a very long way from being worked out and assessed. It should also be obvious that an almost limitless number of different combinations of actions are possible in the respiratory tract during the production of a tone (See Figs. 4, 5, 6 and 7).

Moving the larynx up or down from its position at the bottom of the pharynx also affects timbre, intensity and pitch (See Wyke).[33, 34]

An excellent and more detailed account of these variations in vocal cord movements and configuration, illustrated by photographs and diagrams, is given by Vennard[31] and by Brodnitz[11, 12] and by von Leden.[32]

So far we feel confident in giving certain pieces of advice to a singer, or actor, based directly on the foregoing. We shall refer back to this account in Chapters 4 and 5, and give explanations.

(1) To increase intensity of a given note you must increase breath pressure; but be certain you are also making good use of the augmenting power of your resonators (pharynx and mouth). Great breath pressure is more likely to damage the cords and exhaust the singer or speaker than obtaining the desired intensity as far as possible by resonator action. Also the latter method is more likely to produce a pleasing quality.

(2) Do not attempt to raise pitch ('reach a high note') by greatly increasing breath pressure, or by greatly increasing the muscle action tending to close the glottis, which you can recognize by the sensation known as 'pushing' or 'forcing' a high note, with neck and shoulders stiff and contracted. This is *very* damaging to the cords, and it produces a shrill note. If you cannot reach the desired pitch without using such a method, you are singing too high; the resulting cordal damage is *very* common in operatic tenors and sopranos, who tend to be forced to sing music that is too high for their vocal mechanism. Hence the rule that 'if you cannot sing a high note *softly*, you should not

sing it at all'.

So far the singing of a note has been considered at one instant of time. There must now be added a very important factor that has a marked effect on the sensation produced in the listener and refers to a variation in the attributes of the note from one fraction of a second to another. (For a masterly account of this subject see Bartholomew[1] who describes the high-speed film recording and analysis of sound waves during singing.) This factor is the **vibrato variation** *of intensity, pitch and probably harmonics* that is an essential in the production of a pleasing note. It is very rapid (about six to seven times a second), even, and present in all pleasing voices that were tested by the above worker and by others. At this speed it is not *appreciated* as a variation in pitch, intensity and harmonics (it is not to be confused with the slower and ugly wobble or with the tremolo) but as a pleasant 'richness' of tone.

Now, considering a still longer period of time, during the singing of a *phrase*, certain additional factors come into play:

1. **Articulation** (that is, consonant formation).
2. **Rhythm.**
3. **Flexibility of transition** in changes of pitch, intensity and timbre.

Articulation depends largely on rapid and easy manipulation of tongue, lips and lower jaw. The other two essentials require sure and easy changes of action of all the muscle groups concerned with respiratory, laryngeal and resonator function. Skill results from practice in co-ordinating all these actions, with the avoidance of excessive contractions and the cultivation of smooth and flowing vocal movements.

Though the novice who has read thus far may be depressed, it must be added here that in the trained singer all the above are performed eventually without conscious effort, the mind being left free to consider sentiment and character, and so adapt singing to these that the result is both beautiful and dramatic.

With regard to the production of a note at the larynx, Wyke,[33, 34] from a meticulous series of neurological studies, has concluded that a very short interval of time may be divided into three phases:

1. A pre-phonatory tuning of the laryngeal muscles—which is potentially under conscious, voluntary control.

2. A reflex modulation of the mechanism once the tone is initiated.

3. An acoustic monitoring, which allows the singer to make an additional adjustment if his auditory mechanism so advises.

But though it has been necessary to cover these actions in such detail we can cheer the reader by emphasizing once again that *though breath pressure is under one's conscious control, cord action is only very slightly so and resonator tuning is largely automatic,* the whole being guided by the ear, much as one uses a knife and fork by sight and feel, and not by conscious control of muscles and joints. Almost the only advice directly bearing on this account we have given above, and will discuss more fully in a later chapter; but an incomplete account of these actions would lead to fallacies, and without one the advice could not be shown to rest on sound principles.

We now come to the vexed question of **registers.** As is well known, if a singer, especially if he has had little experience or training, sings a note in the lower part of his range, and from there sings up the scale, there usually occurs one, and frequently two, points where there is a tendency for the voice to 'break.' after which singing up the scale continues in a voice having a different quality (and therefore indicating a readjustment of the vocal mechanism). In a trained singer such 'breaks' are usually smoothed out, there being a more gradual transition from a voice of one general quality to that of another. Thus in most singers two or three different 'voices' can be distinguished, and to these have been given the name **registers.**

The confusion arising on this subject is partly the result of a confused terminology, and partly the fault of those who persist in finding a label for a mechanism they do not understand—and especially when their attention is focused on one or two of many contributory and interrelated actions of, for example, the type mentioned above. As we have tried to emphasize, these actions are numerous, complex, interrelated, and to some extent interdependent; and very few have been worked out or the proportional importance of their individual contributions assessed. The futility, therefore, of referring to the mechanism of production of a particular range of notes by considering just one or two of these many actions should be obvious.

The terminology that has accumulated in this connection has tended to increase with each new invention or method of studying phonation. Thus we may distinguish the period before the vocal cords had been viewed in life; the period immediately after Garcia[15] introduced the laryngoscope which enabled him to see the cords; the years following this when the use of the laryngoscope increased and improvements and different methods of laryngoscopy multiplied; the more recent increase in experimental physics and physiology, and finally the period of high-speed cinematography of the larynx and special radiographic and optical methods (see Brackett[10], Pressman[25], Bellussi and Visendaz[9], Russell and Kennard[28]). All these added to knowledge, but also to terminology, and therefore to confusion.

Terms descriptive of **registers** employed by various authors include: chest, middle and head; long reed and short reed; thick and thin; and more recently by Hollien pulse, modal, loft and flute. In addition much argument has been devoted to the term falsetto register.

Unfortunately the terminology and lack of agreement on this subject has resulted in such confusion that the present author has decided not to add to the length and complexity of a rather elementary book by entering into discussion of this problem.

The quality of tone known as the *covered voice* must be mentioned, however. Bunch[13, 14] recently submitted a number of singers to a panel of judges who, surprisingly, were in agreement as to when each singer was using a *covered* tone. It was then found by radiographic methods that the *covered* quality was produced when the hyoid bone and vocal cords were in a lowered position, usually by one or two centimetres, the soft palate being raised.

It should be added that there is very little difference in the vocal mechanism of *children, men* and *women* except one of *size*. At puberty the male's larynx becomes rather suddenly considerably larger; the female's gradually a little larger. This is sufficient to account for the differences in vocal range. Other changes of growth and age will be dealt with later.

There remain one or two fundamental points concerned with the physics of sound which must be mentioned, for they often cause confusion.

A sound wave travelling through air may be compared to a sea wave travelling towards a watcher on the beach. Each particle of water transmits its momentum to the particle in front of it, but does not itself move appreciably horizontally; thus a log floating in the sea moves upwards and then downwards as the wave passes, but remains approximately over the same point on the sea bed. Converting this into terms of a sound wave from the respiratory tract we may conclude that:

1. The tracheal *air* only progresses to a few inches in front of the face.

2. The resulting *wave*, being transmitted from particle to particle, can travel many yards, at the speed of sound, according to the amplitude of the cordal vibrations, amplification by the resonators, pitch of the note and conditions of the atmosphere and auditorium. On this depends the distance the note can be heard.

3. Though the wave can be to some extent *directed*, according to the direction in which the singer inclines his mouth, *the wave cannot be 'thrown' or 'projected'*. If this be doubted imagine that a singer has recently eaten a peppermint sweet-meat. His unfortunate leading lady may complain of the aroma but it is hardly likely to trouble the conductor of the orchestra—let alone the back row of the gallery, who, it is to be hoped, can hear his voice and must therefore be reached by the sound waves he initiates.

4. The above explains why a good singer need not extinguish a candle flame placed a few inches in front of his mouth.

Another physical point is the difference between *intensity* and *loudness*. The former denotes a physical property of a sound; the latter a degree of stimulus perceived by the auditory apparatus. A person with normal hearing perceives notes of certain pitch ranges as *louder* than those of other pitche ranges, their *intensity* being equal.

In general, voices sound louder as they range from bass, baritone, tenor, contralto, mezzo-soprano to soprano, partly as a result of this phenomenon, and partly because the lowest notes can only be sung comparatively softly for physiological reasons. The bass and lower ranges of the baritone sound especially soft and the higher soprano notes especially loud, but the effect of harmonic partials as well as the fundamental pitch note must be taken into account. Low-pitch organ pipes and piano notes are constructed to sound at high intensities for this reason (see H. Fletcher[2]).

For the sake of completeness, we will merely mention some other factors which certain workers have suggested might possibly be of importance in phonation or song. These possible factors are alteration in the timing of the opening, closing and shut phases of the glottis, consequent upon variations in action of the opening and closing muscles; the possible formation of Æolian or of edge tones, or of combination and difference tones; and the possible action of other vibratile laryngeal structures such as the false cords or the epiglottis (C. and C. L. Jackson[21]). G. O. Russell[28] adds modification by varying consistency and position of pharyngeal walls, by surface noises and by megaphone-like effects. He disagrees with other authors, who apply the term resonance to cover all these actions.

Lastly there is the alleged Bernouille effect, illustrated by blowing between two sheets of paper, which action brings them *together*. The author retains an open mind as to the importance of this phenomenon at the glottis, but recent researchers have given it much emphasis.

3

Attributes Necessary
for Fine Singing

In the previous chapter we described the structure and function of the vocal mechanism without considering in any detail wherein lie the deciding factors which determine whether a particular actor or singer possesses a voice which is *potentially* fine, moderate or poor. It is with these *potentialities* of vocal equipment that we are now concerned; how this equipment may be best employed will be dealt with in the next chapter.

Keeping to our previous division of the vocal organs and bearing in mind the various attributes of tones, phrases and songs which combine to form a singer's performance, we may enumerate the qualities of structure and function necessary for fine singing. These do not greatly differ from those necessary for declamation, save that the actor is allowed discretion in the matter of pitch and pace but less licence with regard to articulation; the absence of music means less demands of volume, but he can be neither helped nor hindered in expression of emotion and rhythm.

The necessary factors present in a *potentially* fine singer, then, are as follows:

1. **'Bellows.'** (a) *Structure.* The larger the air capacity of the lungs the better, that the singer may avoid the necessity for too many breaths, be able to sustain a long phrase without losing control through 'shortness of breath' and to provide sufficient power on occasion for intensities of great volume.

(b) *Function.* No matter how large the chest is, size is of no advantage unless function is satisfactory. The big chest with poor mobility, commonly seen in middle-aged sufferers from asthma-bronchitis, is a poor pair of bellows. The lungs must be capable of rapid filling and a steady, controlled emptying to provide a flow of breath necessary for sustained and controlled song. This requires, therefore, the muscles of the chest wall, diaphragm and upper abdominal wall to be capable of full movement. And apart from poor physique the above may be interfered with as a result of certain diseases, especially by those of the lungs and heart, as well as by advancing age.

Gould and Okamura[16] working in a vocal dynamics laboratory produced convincing evidence that well-trained singers improved their ventilatory capacity, including the controlled function of their abdominal muscles.

2. **Vibrating Folds.** (a) *Structure.* The larynx, and particularly the vocal cords themselves, should be free from damage resulting from disease or injury. Irregularities, thickenings or defects of substance—*especially of the free margins of the cords*—constitute handicaps which, though often surprisingly slight, may be severe. And even if such damage appears to be affecting the quality of the voice but little, its very presence, especially in young singers, calls for a guarded prognosis as to the effect of future years of singing, particularly if the lesion has been produced by persistently improper methods of singing.

Probably for a voice of low tessitura (bass or contralto) a large larynx is necessary, but the converse is *not* true. In fact as far as structure is concerned it is probably true to say that all that is necessary is for the larynx to be of sufficient size and free from disease or injury.

(b) *Function.* The mobile parts of the larynx must be capable of a full range of normal movements. Diseases interfering with these movements, though seen often enough by laryngologists, are comparatively speaking uncommon; their occurrence in a singer usually has a serious effect on the voice—though every laryngologist can recall remarkable exceptions. (The author has recently examined a singer who suffered a recurrent laryngeal nerve paralysis as a result of rheumatic carditis. Although she needed more breath than formerly, she could still sing! Examination revealed that the paralysed cord was nearly in the mid-line and did vibrate on phonation, the still-active cricothyroid muscle and the bilaterally innervated inter-arytenoid muscle allowing sufficient tension and approximation).

In addition to these relatively coarse movements possessed by any healthy larynx, the various muscles regulating the stiffness of the cords, both by stretching and by firming or hardening actions, and also those controlling cord shape and the way in which the two cords' free margins are opposed must be capable of extremely delicate and precise adjustment. Also the glands of the larynx must provide suitable quantities of thin mucus to act as a lubricant of satisfactory consistency for the cords. This important factor of lubrication is often neglected. (See Punt[27] and also Pressman and Keleman[26]). All this is necessary in order that the cords may respond to the air stream in the variable manner outlined in the previous chapter.

3. **Resonators.** *Structure and function* of these cavities must be considered together.

It may be stated at once that the extremely complex problem of resonator function as applied to the voice is very far from being clear. Opinions of various authorities will be given and the present position summarized.

(i) Alex Wood[7] defines *resonance* as the response of a sounding body when its own natural note is played—that is the response of a vibrating system when subjected to a force timed to its own period.

A simple example is to hold a vibrating tuning fork over a tall, wide-mouthed jar which is being silently filled with water; when the water reaches a certain level the note of the fork is heard at greatly increased intensity, indicating that the partly-filled jar now forms a resonator whose natural note is of the same pitch as that of the fork.

Tyndall[6] writing in 1883 noted that if a vibrating tuning fork was held before the mouth and air was breathed through the glottis (without approximating the cords to allow of their vibration) a vowel sound could be produced by adjusting the cavity of the mouth suitably. Other forks produced other vowels.

Helmholtz[4] to whom we owe most of the early research on problems of sound, concluded that voice was the result of fundamental tones and harmonic partials, produced by the vibrating cords, being reinforced by the resonating cavities.

G. O. Russell[28] however, warns against drawing too close an analogy with hollow vessels for each of the former only responds maximally to notes of one pitch, whilst the artist can sing many notes at equivalent intensities without altering his resonating cavities. He also raises the disturbing problem of how a parrot with tiny resonating cavities can become such a good imitator of humans.

(ii) Paget[24] in a well-known work describing a long series of experiments and observations came to the conclusion that larynx sounds are converted into *vowel sounds* by means of double resonance, the larynx sounds being modified first by the pharynx resonator and then by the mouth resonator.

Consonants were similarly formed by changes in resonator action produced by complete or partial closure of the front or back orifice of the front resonator (i.e., the mouth) of the series that produced them.

He also came to various conclusions with regard to human resonator shape and size (some of which are disputed by other authors, as we shall see). Of these we may note:

For maximum *volume* of mouth resonance, the larger it is, and the larger its front orifice is, the better. (However big it is, it is small compared with the wave-length of the vibrations with which we are concerned.) But there is no point in its front orifice being larger than the central dimensions of its cavity. Its back orifice (between mouth and pharynx) should be small.

But the above desiderata with regard to volume must be modified on account of considerations of *pitch*, for the pitch best amplified by a resonator depends on the relation of its volume to its orifice. The *less yielding* the walls of a resonator are, the more efficient it is, but in the case of the mouth firmness of walls must to some extent be sacrificed to flexibility in order to secure more rapid and accurate changes in tuning.

(We would interpolate here that in the case of the pharynx excessive firming of the walls leads to constriction and must be avoided.)

By connecting singers' nostrils to his own ear with a rubber tube Paget noted that several very good singers did not, in the correct physicist's sense, employ nasal resonance when singing. But he suggested that resonation between the back of the tongue and upper part of the soft palate was important at times. Also as a result of his experiments he declared that the nasal sinuses were not important as resonators, that sound inside the mouth cannot be 'thrown' or 'projected,' and that the hard palate and teeth are very much too small to reflect sound waves. (Vibrations of the bones of the skull are, of course, sensed by the *singer*, who hears his voice partly by this bone-conduction. Such sensations may help him, but these vibrations do not contribute to the tones heard by the listener).

(iii) Negus[22, 23] agrees with Paget that a large mouth (and pharynx) are desirable for powerful resonance—and finds support for this contention in his unique series of observations on animals' respiratory tracts. With regard to the position of the larynx as a whole he produces additional evidence in the form of X-ray pictures of a singer to show that a low position of the larynx in the neck, with a capacious pharynx, gives a pleasing timbre, whilst a high position, with a diminished pharynx, results in a tone described as 'throaty'.

He also agrees that the nasal chambers themselves, the sinuses, and the actual larynx cavity have very little resonator action, by reason of their size and position; but opening or closing the naso-pharynx, by means of the soft palate, does have some effect, closure producing 'pure' vowels and opening giving a 'nasal' tone.

Concerning the chest he disagrees with Paget, having formed the opinion that 'the trachea and bronchi, and the air spaces of the lungs, give increase in volume and alteration of quality,' but that they cannot be voluntarily altered in shape and size, merely changing automatically with respiration, and therefore 'act as universal and not as selective resonators'. Our own observations confirm that a big-chested person usually has a correspondingly 'rich, resonant voice'—hence the well-known fact that most fine singers are large-bodied—*but* a big chest usually goes with a big pharynx so the *relative* importance of the chest and pharynx size remains doubtful. Also methods of 'voice production' professing to emphasize 'chest resonance' usually include the maintenance of a low larynx and may insist on absence of pharyngeal constriction, so again the satisfactory 'rich resonance' of the tone may be due to pharyngeal rather than chest resonance.

(iv) Alex Wood[7], in his work on the physics of music, in addition to discussing the various theories already mentioned, gives most interesting tables compounded from scientific

analyses of sung tones; these show very clearly that the differences in timbre between different instruments and voices
depend on which partials are most emphasized, and that any
particular vowel sound, no matter whether sung by bass or
soprano, is recognizable because the predominant partial has a
fixed pitch.

(v) Sundberg[5], in a most interesting series of vocal analyses,
concluded that; 'A man with a wide pharynx and with a larynx
that will resonate at a frequency of between 2500 and 3000
Hertz is likely to be able to develop a good singing voice more
readily than a person who lacks those characteristics. And his
progress may be facilitated if his vocal folds give him a range
that agrees with his formant frequencies. As for a female singer,
she should be able to shift the first formant to join the pitch frequency in the upper part of her range.'

(vi) Bartholomew[1] contributes an extremely important
paper which every singing teacher and all those interested in
the scientific study of singing should read. (It is most readily
available in abstract in the volume by Alex Wood[7]).

The aim of the investigation was to compare physical recordings of æsthetically good and poor voices and to note any
physical differences in the sound waves thus recorded.

With regard to resonance these observations showed that
fine voices were also powerful voices, associated with large
throats, free egress through lower pharynx and over the base of
the tongue (this latter point differs from Paget's opinion) and
greater resonance by tensing of the walls. He also mentions
photographs by Russell indicating that pharyngeal constriction means a poor voice.

In addition he noted that fine male voices showed a
strengthened partial at about 500 cycles and another at about
2400 to 3200 cycles, and that good voices had strong second
partials. The strengthened partials he referred to as a high and
a low *formant*, and their production he presumed to be depen-
dent on resonator action and construction.

He also found (quoting Seashore[50]) remarkably constant in
good singers a smooth *vibrato variation* occurring about six or
seven times a second and affecting pitch, intensity and timbre.
This was *not 'sensed'* as a tremolo or 'wobble,' but as an added
richness of the tone. Its mechanism of production, and even

whether it is a vibrator or resonator effect, is doubtful.

We have discussed this question of resonator structure and function in more detail than that of laryngeal function, the reason being that the various complex laryngeal movements are largely beyond the singer's deliverate control, but adjustment of the size, shape and orifices of the pharynx and mouth, is much more under the singer's direct control, though the *trained* singer should no longer have to think about them, any more than the *expert* horseman thinks about his bodily movements.

We will conclude this consideration of the resonators by summarizing what we consider to be desirable properties of their structure and function for a potentially fine singer. This opinion is based partly on the work of the authors quoted above and partly on our own observations. We do not believe in the present state of our knowledge it is possible to particularize further, when we leave the laboratory behind and come to consider individual singers.

(i)   The chest, pharynx and mouth should be large, and

(ii) they should be free from disease or injury.

(iii) The muscular components of the pharynx and mouth—and especially the tongue and soft palate (see Fig. 1)—must be capable of rapid and controlled mobility, without excessive contraction.

(iv) The parts concerned must be appropriately lubricated with adequate quantities of thin mucus or saliva.

(v)   There should be no condition causing irritation of the mucous membrane, and no muscle should be put under so much tension that it leads to a sensation of aching or tiredness in the throat or neck during the course of an evening's singing. In fact singing should not cause any feeling of discomfort, unless indulged in to excess or rôles are attempted for which the singer's vocal mechanism or training makes him unsuited.

(vi) The resonators—particularly the pharnyx and mouth—should be so *fortunately constituted* with regard to dimensions, orifices and properties of their walls that their influence on larynx notes is greatly to augment their volume. At the same time they should emphasize certain harmonic partials so as to achieve beauty and richness of timbre, clarity of words, and colour or expression varying appropriately to accord with and enrich the sentiments and emotions embodied in the opera or other work. We do not believe our knowledge at present permits of any precise description of what these dimensions should be ideally, nor what dimensional relations one resonator should bear to another.

This would seem an appropriate place to discuss a question constantly in the minds of operatic directors, impresarios and others whose life is much taken up with the search for fine voices—and especially for young, little-known singers who possess the potentialities described above, and can be trained to fulfil their particular requirements in opera, oratorio or concerts as the case may be.

'*Why are voices of great power and beautiful timbre so scarce?*' Many will give reasons associated with fashion and taste or with changing habits and customs, but these are only subsidiary factors. Most purveyors of a method, system or theory of singing will declare that if only *they* were to be entrusted with the training of young singers, Carusos and Melbas would soon abound. But they never do, no matter how many students they attract, how well they are advised, or how assiduously they study! The fact is that singing is *not* a natural act, but an accomplishment as artificial as juggling and more so than acrobatics. (The singing of birds is by a rather different mechanism.) The most convincing evidence for the unnaturalness of singing as the term is generally understood is provided by Negus[22, 23] in his observations of the manner in which the human larynx has evolved from those of the animal kingdom; speech, even, is evolutionally speaking a very late function of the larynx (see Chapter 8).

Potentially fine voices, therefore, are unusual accidents of Nature, and really great voices might fairly be described as freaks.

And when in addition one considers that such a vocal mechanism may chance to be possessed by a person of any walk of life, that such a person may never find his way into musical circles, that if he does he may be taken up by a singing teacher whose methods ruin his larynx, that defects of hearing, personality, character, intellect or intelligence may prove fatal to his training or career—then we need not wonder that great voices employed for our delight by great artists are so rare as to be phenomenal.

The emotional make-up or temperament of the artist, without which the mechanism is uninspired and useless, has been discussed in Chapter 1.

Having enumerated as precisely as possible the factors necessary for a potentially fine voice, we must now consider how these properties of structure and function may best be assessed in individual would-be singers. It is to be feared that many whose duty it is to select students likely to benefit by singing training, or directors of opera searching for fresh voices for their companies, would answer simply 'let them sing a few songs or arias and listen!' The disadvantages of employing this method exclusively are twofold. Firstly, defects of voice may be due to poor training, and not to deficiencies of vocal mechanism. Contrariwise, a young singer at an audition may exhibit a voice of such power, range and timbre that a successful career is immediately prophesied; but if the effect is achieved by methods damaging to the vocal mechanism the career will be a short one.

Having, then, described the various factors necessary for a potentially fine voice, we will now suggest how the presence or absence of these potentialities may be *assessed*. We will consider the example of a young man who has had some training but little experience, and presents himself as a candidate for a position in an opera company, hoping that continuance of training and the singing of chorus of minor parts will eventually lead to principal rôles.

A laryngologist accustomed to singers and actors will know at once that his patient is suffering from some degree of anxiety and may even be terrified, although he may try to disguise his emotions by a display of bravado or indifference. He is hoping for reassurance, and for praise of his vocal mechanism and abilities. He may ask whether one can assess his vocal potentialities by examining his throat, in which case he must be told that defects are often easily detected (and may sometimes be remedied) but that potential abilities, even in a splendidly healthy and well-constructed throat, will only be revealed in the course of time. When one has unhurriedly established an atmosphere of mutual trust, confidence and understanding, having listened patiently to everything the aspirant has to say, he is examined with particular attention to the following details:

1. Has he a large healthy **chest,** and can he fill his lungs rapidly with air and control their emptying?

2. (a) Does examination with the laryngeal mirror reveal a **larynx** free from disease and injury, with an apparently full range of movements?

(b) Does the laryngeal mucus appear normal in consistency and quality?

(c) Continued research may eventually enable one conveniently to record the nature of cord vibrations—especially by such means as ultra slow-motion photography and fibre-optical equipment, but at the time of writing the complex, expensive and largely experimental apparatus is available only at a few laboratories, and interpretation of the records is still speculative. Violins and organs differ, but merely looking at them will only reveal comparatively gross defects.

3. (a) Has he a large **pharynx** and **mouth**?

(b) Are the mobile structures of his pharynx and mouth capable of full movement, and are they free from disease or injury?

(c) Are these parts satisfactorily lubricated?

(d) Are the **nose** and **sinuses** healthy, and the teeth and gums well cared for?

4. Has he good **hearing?** The usual examination familiar to otologists may be necessary.

5. Finally, does he appear generally **healthy** and **robust?** Contrary to popular impression, the life of an actor or singer is a hard one physically and exhausting emotionally. Poor health and physique may be overcome by the indomitable spirit possessed by so many theatre-folk—an inflexible determination and courage that makes an actor go on to play his part though he feels, and indeed may be, at the point of death, and which no one ignorant of the atmosphere of the theatre can understand. But if such handicaps are detected in the young, and especially if no great abilities or potentialities are apparent, it is kindest to dissuade such an aspirant at the outset. (Not that one ever can!)

To summarize the information obtainable by such an examination, one may conclude that only *defects* can be accurately judged; and these generally reveal themselves as evidence of disease or injury, or a lack of a vocal mechanism of sufficient size. *Particularly note that to try to make a Grand Opera singer of a slightly built, small-throated, narrow-chested individual, no matter how healthy, or how attractive the little voice sounds in a drawing-room, is as futile as trying to obtain notes of Cathedral organ quality from a small harmonium. And the attempt will ruin the larynx irreparably and be the cause of heartache and suffering in one who, properly advised, might have a profitable and artistic career as a ballad singer or in operetta or musical comedy.*

The above details of structure and function, and of health, having been noted we may now allow the aspirant to sing. There have been several attempts to classify voices: Walshe[55] awarded 'marks' for certain named qualities of 'voice, vocalization and dramatic expression'. Moses[47] defined what he described as 'acoustic dimensions'. Seashore[50] was careful to differentiate between a singer's appreciation of various properties of sound and his ability to reproduce the desirable properties in his own voice. He also assessed 'musical memory, imagination, intellect and intelligence'; but in our opinion his most valuable service has been to produce evidence showing which of these properties are largely *inherited* (and therefore if a young singer does not possess them, no amount of training will impart them) and which can be *acquired* or improved with training. Those interested are advised to read his book for a fascinating account of the researches by which he reached these conclusions.

Field-Hyde[42] in his book on voice training gives details of charts he has devised to record the various attributes of his pupils' voices. The use of such records, being the singing teacher's equivalent of the doctor's case notes, must be of great value, and the pupil's progress can be readily studied with their aid.

The degree and nature of improvement to be expected from continued training and experience in a young singer is often a difficult matter to assess. Schatz[49] made the dogmatic and provocative statement that most good singers give evidence of their exceptional voice before they meet a voice trainer. Seashore[50] concluded that a sense of appreciation of pitch, intensity, time, rhythm and possibly timbre were inherited; but that in a singer who *had* inherited such a well-marked sense of appreciation, training could to a variable degree improve the quality of these attributes in his own performance. On the other hand if he lacked the sense of appreciation of these attributes, he was unable to acquire them, and consequently unable to improve his singing—presumably because he could not detect his own defects. This seems to be borne out by experience; a tone-deaf person cannot be taught to discriminate between sounds of slightly different pitch, nor can one inculcate an appreciation of rhythm or of timbre in one markedly lacking such senses. Semon's[29] experience was in accord with these findings. But probably few people with such a sadly defective sensorium persist with their training beyond an elementary stage. Endeavours to obtain evidence on these points from such sources as biographies of fine singers are rather more entertaining than helpful. Such evidence drawn from books by Tetrazzini[54] (mentioning Caruso, Jenny Lind and Pasta), by Fucito[44] (Caruso's coach and accompanist), by Diana Tauber[79] and by many others is conflicting.

Oren Brown,[37] a fine and dedicated teacher of the Juilliard School of Music, New York, summarised his many years of experience thus: 'In the clinical situation (*e.g.*, a voice studio) all other examinations are supplemented by the eye and ear of one sensitized by broad experience. Tessitura, hypo- or hyperfunction, and type of rôle being performed need to be evaluated against the optimum potential of the artist's voice (range and size) and his habitual speech patterns. One must also be aware of such factors as empathy, sympathy, register adjustments, and vowel modification.'

To return to our singer, when the laryngologist has finished his examination. Then the director of the opera company should be willing to hear him sing. Bearing in mind the various types of singing for which the aspirant's voice may be found suitable, attention should be paid to the following points, being particularly careful in the case of an inexperienced singer to consider *potentialities, whether any defects may be remedied by training, and whether the singer can only obtain his effects by methods liable to damage his larynx.*

1. **Intensity.** If the voice is not 'big' enough it is no use for 'big' operatic rôles—no matter how beautiful it is, how wide its range and expression or how attractive the singer. If he has not been endowed with a vocal mechanism capable of producing his range of tones with sufficient volume and without forcing, every effort should be made to dissuade him from attempting such rôles. If the opera director or singing teacher allows himself to be blinded to lack of this essential by the presence of other qualities, he will be responsible for the ruin of a voice, and of a career which properly directed might have been artistically and financially successful. This is a common tragedy. (But that is not to say that he must sing at full volume all the time. Far from it! Much singing, and especially tenors' and sopranos' high notes, should often be quite soft, but the volume should be obtainable when required.)

2. **Pitch.** (a) *Compass and Tessitura.* Probably the majority of English male voices are most suitable for training as baritones, and most female as mezzo-sopranos; the highest notes demanded of an operatic tenor or soprano are certainly too high for the vast majority of singers to attain without some degree of strain (see Chapters 4 and 5). Unfortunately the demand is largely for such sopranos and tenors, partly because these voices have greatest appeal and so many fine rôles have been written for them, and partly for this very reason—that their scarcity tempts operatic directors to entrust such parts to vocally ill-equipped singers, who do not last long as a result. Having decided the compass of the voice and its range (we suspect too often the mere 'possession' of high notes is emphasized), particular attention should be focused on whether the high notes can be produced without employing a method liable to damage the voice.

(b) *Accuracy of Pitch.* If the singer is habitually liable to sing off-pitch the fault is probably an inherited defect of pitch judgment and little can be done about it. An instrument that might be more widely used is the tonoscope by which the singer can see, by watching the instrument as he sings, how accurately he keeps to pitch (see Alex Wood[7], Harvey Fletcher[2] and Seashore[50]).

3. **Timbre.** (*a*) If a singer is able to produce notes of sufficient range and volume, he is likely to obtain some measure of
success. But unless the tones of his voice have also a beauty of
timbre over a considerable part of his range he will never rouse
a critical audience to enthusiasm. Some physical properties of
sound waves repeatedly found to be present in singers with
beautiful voices have been mentioned in the previous chapter,
and the little information available concerning the probable
factors influencing the production of these characteristics has
been given. But however far scientists may progress in relating
beauty of timbre to overtone structure and vibrato variations,
evaluation of such beauties will remain a matter of sensory appreciation largely unconnected with intellect, intelligence and
scientific knowledge.

(*b*) While assessing these qualities it may become apparent
that the voice is suitable for a certain *range of parts*. No artist is so
versatile as to be able to embody characters expressing every
possible variation of emotion. Consequently the singer should also
be judged with regard to his ability to adapt his tone quality and
expression in accordance with sentiment and character. In a young
singer much may be hoped for as a result of training in this
necessity: much, but not too much.

Sopranos and tenors are often described as being either
'lyric' or 'dramatic'. We are afraid the first designation usually
implies a voice which is lovely, but light; and the second one
which is powerful, but impressive rather than beautiful. The
great voice is both, but these being scarce phenomena the terms
have their uses when classifying voices of less splendour.

(*c*) Finally some estimation should be attempted on the
probable effect on the voice of increasing *age*.

4. **Breath Control.** Given the necessary physique this is largely a matter of training, and is absolutely essential for fine
singing. Few things are more distressing to behold than a singer
obviously troubled by inability to obtain sufficient breath to
sustain long phrases or negotiate rapid passages. It is only too
obvious that this consideration is preventing the singer from
concentrating on beauty and appropriateness of tone and
rhythm, and instead of listening in sympathy to the character

our feelings are diverted to sympathy for the singer and blame for the management that permits such agonizing.

5. **Rhythm, and flexibility and smoothness of transition** in changes of pitch, intensity and timbre.

These necessary accomplishments are also largely matters of training, but if found to be gravely defective it should be ascertained whether there is an inherited, irremedial lack of appreciation of these essentials.

6. **Articulation.** We must admit to a personal bias on this point. Most opera lovers are either not interested in 'hearing the words' or else know them so well as to be able to supply them from memory. We prefer to be able to hear them. The difficulty is that a soprano's high notes cannot for physical reasons contain sufficient low resonances for her to articulate at all clearly whilst singing them. Other female singers, and tenors, are troubled to a varying extent. In addition, English and German contains so many closures (e.g., S, Z, J, X, ch and sh) that they are very difficult to sing understandably, whilst French and, especially, Italian are full of open vowels and are, as is well known, easier to sing in consequence. Our own preference would be to insist that singers pay more attention to articulation, but allow them to sing Italian and French works in their original languages. This having been said, articulation is also largely a matter of training, and of emphasizing the bite of certain consonants.

It is also noteworthy that a singer who finds it difficult to enunciate words clearly is often attempting parts beyond her capabilities, and is thus so hard put to it to sing the music at all that attention to words is impossible. This is most commonly found with sopranos, and some composers and librettists, knowing this, are careful to entrust important details of plot to voices of lower *tessitura*.

7. **Style and Personality** together with appearance and acting ability should be noted. Too many singers possess a voice and little else. Judging from theatrical history, only Chaliapin (and possibly Caruso) would appear to have earned the dual title of great singer and fine actor. A particular difficulty

concerning those who aspire to playing romantic rôles concerns the question of figure. As we have shown, the possessor of a big voice must be well built—not necessarily fat, as unkind legend would have it, but of such a size as to make the impersonation of many romantic rôles an embarrassment. Clearly nothing can be done about this, but the acquisition of acting ability should not be neglected, nor the cultivation of an individual style and exploitation of personality. What can be expected from training and experience in any particular case requires experienced judgment.

8. **Intelligence and Character.** Some estimation of these may be made at this interview, allowing for nervousness and the effort to create a good impression, both as regards affairs of general conduct and concerning musical matters. Such factors, apart from singing ability, have to be considered in casting an opera or deciding a singer's rôles for a coming season.

Though not a usual practice in this country, it would seem to us an excellent thing to complete this assessment of potentialities by making some attempt at correlation of the laryngologist's findings and the opera director's, especially to determine whether a laryngological reason could be found for any fault in a student's singing. But it is, of course, essential that any such three-cornered consultation should be with the full approval of the singer, who would still be able to entrust future confidences to the laryngologist, the latter's first duty remaining always to his patient.

4
Care and Use of the Voice in Health

'The number of muscles controlling the respiratory organs is considerable, when consideration is given to those of the mouth, lower jaw, tongue, soft palate, pharynx, hyoid apparatus, larynx, neck, thorax and abdominal wall; it is not surprising, therefore, to find enormous individual variations in the control of the voice, since management of this team of muscles, only partly under the influence of the higher cerebral centres, is difficult to attain. In addition, variations in the size and shape of the resonators add further complexity. The teaching of singing is therefore a matter of difficulty, and one depending mainly on empirical factors' (Negus[22]).

In this chapter we shall endeavour to define certain principles which should be observed in order to employ the vocal mechanism in such a way as to produce the finest effects of which it is capable, but without damaging the parts concerned in structure or function. *No more than this is attempted.* We do not usurp the function of the singing teacher, nor advocate any theory or method of singing, but merely state what little can be learnt from anatomy and from physiological and physical laws which appears to be of value to singers and their teachers. In the next chapter we make some endeavour to correlate neglect of these principles with vocal defects and laryngeal damage. This determination to keep as far as possible to facts which can be supported by evidence explains, and we hope excuses, a lack of completeness about this chapter. It is easy enough to sit in an armchair with pencil, paper and a few books and concoct a 'theory of singing'. It is easier still for the uncritically and unscientifically minded, with the help of a picturesque jargon, to delude themselves into believing that their pupils' vocal organs are being trained to act in accordance with this theory; and, given sufficient personality and a few potentially good voices, their students—usually completely without scientific training and with critical faculties undeveloped—readily believe this too. Eventually they bring their damaged larynges for inspection, chattering the while in this same jargon. Some of the more popular or publicized of these theories will be dealt with in the last chapter. We will content ourselves now with simply requesting the reader to bear in mind the main particulars we have outlined concerning the structure and function of the vocal mechanism, and to consider critically the precise meaning of every term and statement applied to singing in relation to these basic facts. Far better to say, 'we do not know,' admitting gaps in our understanding, than to fill these in with vague or ill-considered notions having little or no evidence in their support.

Even fine singers seldom have scientifically unassailable views of these matters; perusal of their writings will confirm this; and likewise that there exists a complete lack of agreement even over terminology. Shakespeare[51] in one of the better books on singing, summarizes the advice of several singers, including many old masters, and again we note this divergence of views, and terminology more picturesque than precise. Study of singers' biographies will readily reveal the chaos resulting from the number of academies professing to teach particular methods of singing in various parts of the world. A good example, chosen almost at random, is the autobiography of Lotte Lehmann[77].

The suggestions we have to make concerning the use of the voice will now follow, together with evidence in their support and reasons that lead to these conclusions. We have not found it possible to achieve any systematic order—indeed we are not sure that such an endeavour might not be a source of error, for it is important when studying individual singers to consider the vocal mechanism not only as regards its separate organs, but as a whole—the actions of groups of muscles in one region, for example, may be related to those in another. There will therefore be some unavoidable overlapping with the succeeding chapter, but a certain amount of such repetition may not be a bad thing.

1. **Avoid 'glottic shock' ('coup de glotte').** (*a*) There are two main sets of factors causing the vocal cords to resist the onward passage of the tracheal air-stream: the first is the variable stiffness of the cords themselves; the second is the force of the sphincteric group of muscles tending to oppose the cords and thus close the glottis (see Figs. 5, 6 and 7). The more powerfully these two groups of muscles contract (the 'closing' group and the 'stiffening' group) the higher the pitch of the note formed when the air pressure does overcome this resistance and thus set the cords vibrating. If this resistance is mainly due to cord stiffness no harm is done to the cord's surface; but if to obtain the desired high note the singer excessively increases the power of the sphincteric closing muscles, then the vibrating cords are, in fact, opposed and consequently strike against one another inflicting damage each to the other—resulting in the so-called singers' or screamers' nodes, nodules, corns, warts or vocal nodules of attrition. This we believe to be the mechanism of the *coup de glotte*, which produces these nodules.

We would like to be able to prove the above contention, but doubt whether it is susceptible of complete proof. However, we believe it to be in accordance with physical and physiological facts. Over the years the author has collected a series of colour transparencies of microscopic sections of vocal nodules which he has removed. They are in varying stages of development (as subdivided in Chapter 5) and their appearances correlate well with the patients' vocal histories.

Observation, by ourselves and others, shows that these nodules occur about the mid-point of the membranous cords, consequently about where the vibratory swing would be likely to cause the cords to strike one another, and that there is an association between the glottic shock method of attack and the production of these nodules. We would add that there seems to be no other method by which the cords could be so damaged, than by this striking one against the other.

(*b*) Probably most singers reading these words will recognize the type of attack to which we have been referring. Typically, the singer achieves a high note by greatly tensing all her throat and often neck muscles, increasing breath pressure, and then allowing the breath to burst through the glottis. The result, at its worst, is a shrill shriek delivered by a soprano with tense neck, swelling veins and empurpled face. The groundlings may enjoy their astonishment; the judicious grieve; and we wonder when the poor girl will be along to ask for a throat spray and tell us her notions of 'voice production'!

(*c*) Such a catastrophic manoeuvre can be avoided, at least during practice, by singing scales on open vowels such as MA, MAW or FAH, rather than on EE, thus preventing 'glottic shock'.

(*d*) Don't raise breath pressure to achieve a high note.

(*e*) Sing most high notes softly, and practise tapering off to a diminuendo, rather than swelling to the crescendo of which you are so proud.

(*f*) Singing legato (that is smoothly, without breaks, flowing) is much less harmful to the larynx than staccato methods, which should therefore be avoided except when the score compels. One has heard staccacto passages which represented a series of glottic shocks. Sopranos are frequent offenders.

2. **Avoid excessive muscular contraction** especially of the throat and neck muscles.

(*a*) Certain groups of muscles tend to act together. In singing, such groups are the sphincteric closing muscles of the glottis, the sheet-like muscles in the walls of the pharynx, and certain neck muscles including those which pull the larynx as a whole upwards. Consequently if one of these muscle groups is put into strong contraction (such as the sphincteric, closing group in glottic shock) the other groups contract too. As a result the pharynx becomes constricted and the larynx rises as a whole. Bartholomew[8], in a characteristically excellent article, states that the aim of the singing teacher should be to obtain in his pupil a 'large, relaxed, low throat' in order to secure good resonance. This is why singing teachers get good results by 'taking the pupil's mind off the throat' and talking of 'opening the throat,' 'head resonance,' 'singing in the masque' and other useful, but fanciful, imageries. Oren Brown,[37] in a recent seminar, made the excellent declaration that 'a voice should grow to its own potential'.

(*b*) In addition to impaired resonation, such overaction of muscles will lead to a lack of motility of tongue, lips and cheeks.

It will also cause a sensation of aching and tiredness in the muscles of the throat and neck. This is a very frequent complaint, and its mode of production is not dissimilar to that of aching in muscle groups of the arms and legs as a result of excessive exercise. *Unfortunately* the more delicate muscles controlling laryngeal action do not ache appreciably, and it is not till the larger pharynx and neck muscles are affected that the singer is warned. By this time the larynx muscles have probably been considerably overworked—to which they may react by suddenly failing to respond at all to a closing or firming impulse. We have known this happen in the middle of a performance. (It must be very carefully distinguished from loss of voice due to 'nervous' cases.) Such a sudden inability to sing occurring during the course of an opera has a petrifying effect on the singer, and a peculiar reaction on the company. The unfortunate victim must be treated with extreme care, physically and psychologically.

(*c*) Some tenors achieve high notes by firmly opposing the rear portions of their vocal cords, thus shortening the anterior vibrating portions, and so raising pitch. This is known as arytenoid stop-closure. We regard it as a legitimate manoeuvre as long as the posterior closure is not too forceful, in which case the posterior arytenoid area of the vocal cords may suffer damage.

3. **Only Sing Roles within your** *tessitura*. (*a*) As has been said, the highest pitches demanded of operatic tenors and sopranos cannot be achieved, except in rare instances, without causing the vocal mechanism to act in a forcible manner which is liable to injure the larynx. Unfortunately this has been neglected by composers, and the luckless singers have no alternative but to sing these notes as best they can. This is one reason why laryngeal damage is so much more commonly seen in these classes of singers, as any laryngologist can confirm. So strongly did Cathcart[39]—himself a singers' laryngologist of repute—feel about this, that when he helped to finance the first Promenade Concerts at the Queen's Hall in 1894 he insisted that 'the orchestral instruments should be tuned to French pitch and not to the higher concert pitch, as was then usual'.

With regard to musical directors, we can confirm that singers will be lucky to get much help from them. Alfred Alexander[36] makes it clear that to many conductors the singers are somewhat of a nuisance, whom they would prefer to regard as merely instrumentalists employed to contribute to what they regard as *their* interpretation of an Opera.

The authors findings agree with those of C. and C. L. Jackson[59, 60] who noted that: vocal nodules are commonest in sopranos, next so in tenors, and deplore the fact that 'most of a soprano's professional career, unfortunately, is devoted to extending her range upwards'. We would add that many sopranos find that they can only reach the desired high notes with sufficient volume by employing the glottic shock attack; hence the nodules, as we have explained. The remedy is either to give up the more exacting dramatic rôles, or to give up Grand Opera entirely, or to find out whether after all the voice is not best suited to the mezzo-soprano range. Unfortunately none of this advice is ever received cheerfully by such a singer; ambition and the demand for sopranos militate against its acceptance. But we would sooner meet a happy mezzo than a sad soprano!

We would again emphasize that if you cannot sing a high note softly, you ought not to sing it at all—or at the most only a few notes a week. Loud high notes at full pressure are, to say the least, potentially injurious.

Of course we realize that such advice if really strictly followed would lead to some large gaps in opera repertoires. We cannot help this. We are trying to help and advise singers. Heaven knows they need it! The reader who understands no more of the stage than he learns from his stall and by reading his newspaper sees nothing of the tragedy of ruined voices and frustrated hopes. We do. And we know what mad things a young singer will do to play a coveted part—with the connivance of a manager at his wits' end to find voices that can encompass popular operatic parts at salaries that will not bankrupt his company.

(*b*) The problem of *tessitura* or vocal range is less serious in other types of voice, though one occasionally sees baritones do themselves harm by posing as basso profundos—actually a very rare voice, though most bass-baritones can manage it occasionally without much harm. Caruso, even, is said to have sung the famous bass aria in Bohème in an emergency!

A valuable guide, though not strictly applicable to sopranos, is that of the famous Lamperti who, according to Tetrazzini[54], judged not only by the notes that could be sung, but by those on which words could be enunciated.

Vocal range in a beginner can be determined only as training progresses, and we would stress that only notes which can be sung without excessive muscular contraction, and with volume and timbre under perfect control, should be considered as properly within that singer's range.

(c) Much has been written about 'use of the registers,' and we have explained how this subject has become so confused. It seems to us clear that if a singer finds it necessary to make a change in the mode of action of his vocal mechanism as he ascends the scale, such change should be as gradual as possible. As previously stated, we will leave this vexed question to teachers of singing—with the hope that one day they will make a start at putting their house in order by, at least, coming to some agreement as to terminology.

(d) Carefully-used voices mature with age. When the youthful tones of a Romeo or a Juliet have inevitably been lost, the fuller, more authoritative qualities needed for an Othello or a Lady Macbeth may be achieved. To produce a performance at a drama or singing school the older, dominant rôles may have to be entrusted to young players, and the director may feel this is a valuable part of their education. But this practice is often dangerous to the larynx and we view it with apprehension. The converse may apply; there comes a time when the silver voiced Hamlet is no more, and the player's more discerning admirers wish him to lay the part aside. Moreover, the older artist may damage his larynx if he now has to strain for the higher-pitched vocal passages. It is far better to move on to rôles more suited to the maturer voice, and it is a matter for delight that the truly fine artist, who never stops learning, can produce qualities of voice as the years pass which astonish even those who have closely followed his career. A good account is given by Perello.[64]

(e) A few words should be said about children's voices. The *tessitura* of the child's voice is higher than that of the adult because his larynx is smaller. Its volume is less, because his bellows are less powerful and his vibrator and resonators smaller.

At puberty, as a result of the action of certain glandular secretions, boys' larynges become suddenly larger. For a time there is a lack of control over the voice—which is said to be 'breaking'. Then the voice becomes again controllable, but deeper in pitch. The change in girls is less marked and more gradual. Finally chest, throat and mouth enlarge with bodily growth, the voice becoming louder, and richer in timbre. Training in any branch of music before puberty should discover to what extent a sense of *appreciation* of musical qualities and attributes is present, and should also reveal any musical interest, liking or intellect. To that extent such training may be valuable, and actual training in singing may possibly contribute. But even in the unlikely event of a boy's or girl's teacher giving well-founded advice, we doubt very much if this training is going to be of real value should the pupil eventually study to become an adult professional singer. Nor does the quality of the child's voice enable one to foretell with any accuracy what it will become in later years. Any value such training may have is more likely to be psychological—getting the child used to singing and musical surroundings before the age when he is likely to be made self-conscious thereby. This latter applies even more to the art of acting.

In practice the tendency is for children with beautiful voices to be exploited—by proud parents, by managers and by choirmasters, who should know better. The delicate, still-growing, vocal mechanism is subjected to most of the insults we have been describing—especially singing in the wrong *tessitura* and the various types of forcing—and the larynx is ruined. It is a sad thing to see nodules on the cords of a boy soprano, whose fond mother imagines he has a great and profitable career ahead of him.

Our advice is to regard children's singing entirely as a recreation and, if desired, a method of discovering any inherited musical *appreciation*. The advice in these pages on the care of the voice should be particularly strictly followed; and if it is suspected that the slightest harm is being done to the larynx by over-use or by improper methods of singing, appropriate action should be taken. These remarks apply as much to church singing as to any other form of singing.

Serious training of the voice for professional purposes,

therefore, should not begin till after puberty. Semon[29] says the age of 16 years is early enough. And, of course, whilst the voice is actually 'breaking' singing must be forbidden.

At one time castration used to be performed on boy singers. This prevented the laryngeal enlargement associated with puberty, but not generally bodily enlargement, including chest and pharynx. Consequently these eunuchs sang with a boy's *tessitura* but with greater volume and probably a richer timbre. We still have music written for castrati and such rôles are sometimes attempted by modern 'falsetto tenors'. This may be the cause of trouble, and we cannot but think it unwise (see Negus[23] and a most interesting historical account by Brodnitz).[12]

4. **Do not Sing too Loud or too Often.** (*a*) The various muscles which control the laryngeal form and movements are small and delicate, especially those situated within the substance of the vocal cord itself. If, for example, the muscles of a limb are exercised too violently or for too long they begin to ache. We have been warned to rest. Most *unfortunately* no such warning ache occurs in these small larynx muscles, as it may in the throat and neck. Consequently the singer may employ these too violently (e.g. by singing too loudly or at too high pitches) and for too long. The first laryngeal warning is a 'weakness' or 'hoarseness' of the voice, due to the tired laryngeal muscles failing in their firming, thinning or opposing actions on the cords. Like the limb muscles, the treatment is rest, followed by resumption of *gentle* exercise—i.e. *silence*, followed by a *gentle* resumption of speaking and singing. Such over-use continued for years leads to a permanent weakness of the muscles concerned. C. Jackson and C. L. Jackson[59, 60] named this myasthenia of the larynx. We cannot do better than quote from their excellent writings:

'Practically all singers eventually ruin their voices because of the unnatural and always excessive singing and vocal exercising in which they are required to indulge. No matter how good the quality of the voice may be as a natural endowment, it constitutes only a good instrument; to develop a great artistic result requires many years of practice on that instrument. This training ruins almost all voices.

'. . . the work of the professional teacher of vocal music. He does not understand that the condition is one of overwork of the larynx; and, moreover, he does not understand that overwork and over-exercise do not strengthen the muscles but increase their feebleness. It is true that the athletic coach enormously increases the muscular power of the athlete by severe and prolonged training; but it is equally true that any attempt to do the same thing with the larynx almost invariably results in a progressive weakening of the muscles and eventual ruin of their power. Not understanding this, the vocal teacher is constantly devising some new exercise or some new method of singing or of laryngeal control to cure this form of hoarseness; the result is increasing hoarseness and utter ruin of the larynx for professional vocalization.'

Particularly rest the voice as much as possible when there is any throat inflammation, discomfort or sensation of tiredness. Do not force it all the harder.

We shall return to this subject in Chapters 5 and 6.

(*b*) To summarize, avoid over-use of the voice by singing *too often* at performance, practice or rehearsal; or by singing *too loudly*, especially the higher notes. Too-heavy rôles must be firmly refused, and singing should be avoided in halls having poor acoustics, or in the open air, where the singer does not get his own voice reflected back to him, cannot judge volume accurately, and therefore tends to exceed.

In addition, avoid over-use of the voice on *social occasions*, and especially in noisy surroundings, such as at parties or when travelling.

First-Night parties are a particular menace. We often tell a player that we will get him through his First Night, but that if he spends more than five minutes at the party afterwards, there won't be much of a second night! This injunction is usually obeyed, but we have seen it ignored and have had to cope with consequent damage.

5. **Breathe without undue Constriction or Discomfort.**
(*a*) We do not intend to spend much time on this extremely vexed question, for we believe that a lot of rather pointless argument has arisen in the past without any satisfactory conclusion,

and doubt very much if a great deal can be learned from reading about breathing anyway.

Froeschels[43] tested eight prominent singers and found that, each of them breathed differently!

Further reference may be made to writings of Cathcart[39], Browne and Behnke[38], Shakespeare[51], Holbrook Curtis[41], Moses[47], Guthrie[17, 46], Aikin[35], Hemery[18] and Field-Hyde[42].

As Oren Brown stated in a recent Seminar, 'a singer is an expert professional breather'.

(*b*) In brief, release of breath during production of a phrase is controlled by muscles of the walls of the abdomen and chest, the diaphragm being in relaxation. Attempting to gain additional breath and control by raising the collar-bones and accentuating movements of the upper chest is a fault. Such an endeavour tends to cause constriction of the tongue and neck; no animal employs such a method when it requires extra breath (Negus[22]).

6. **Articulate as Clearly as Possible.** We have explained why it is difficult to articulate clearly when singing, especially in English and German, and would merely emphasize that it is the singer's duty to do his best when the demands of music allow.

7. **Colour your tones appropriately** to the sentiment and emotion you are expressing.

(*a*) This, too, we have emphasized elsewhere. The aim of the singer should be to attain such technical assurance that singing is performed almost automatically, the mind being free to dwell on the appropriate emotion and colour to be related to words and phrases.

The singer acts with his voice, but 'keeps a critical fraction of himself free from absorption in the part played' (Hemery[18]).

Sing with a cool head and a warm heart (Caruso[74]).

Plunket Greene's[45] book 'Interpretation in Song' expresses clearly what should be the aims which a singer should strive to attain.

(*b*) If *you* feel convinced that you have a beautiful voice, but *others* deny this, the fault may be that the voice sounds richer to you than to your audience because one hears one's own voice partly by conduction through the bones of the head, which alters the character of the sound-pattern actually received by the inner ear. The answer is to have recordings made. A good electric-tape recorder* which can be at once played back is excellent. You can then really hear yourself as others hear you. Aim always at *beauty* of timbre if you would delight, rather than astonish, your audience.

(*c*) Field-Hyde[42] in his book on voice training gives an interesting chart showing the use he makes of the different vowels in singing scales in order to develop particular tone-colours in his pupils; but that is the singing teacher's affair, as long as he is careful in permitting use of the dangerous E.

(*d*) We have mentioned articulation and appropriate tone colour in this section because we believe that ability to pay attention to these factors indicates that shocks and strains of the vocal mechanism are being as far as possible avoided. Shrill, harsh or throaty singers, whose words are indistinguishable, usually have poor control over the vocal mechanism. Tones which cause no discomfort to the singer, and sound mellow and beautiful to the listener, are seldom produced by shocking the glottis or putting unnecessary strain on throat muscles.

8. **Avoid as far as possible risking damage to the throat by:**

(*a*) Over-use of tobacco and alcohol; or breathing harmful atmospheres such as those vitiated by dusts, tobacco smoke, car exhaust fumes, etc. Be wary of home decorating; paint fumes are often harmful to the throat. Also avoid poorly ventilated rooms and, especially in America, buildings with excessively warming and drying heating systems ('desiccating', Jackson[59, 60] calls them.) Efficient humidifiers are now available, and some are portable.

(*b*) Exposure to cold, wet or foggy weather.

(*c*) Excessively cold or hot foods and drinks.

(*d*) Harmful sprays, paints or gargles.

In conclusion one must say a word about broadcasting and

---

*Mr. Ernest Newman, writing in the *Sunday Times* of August 12th, 1951, notes with approval that 'Bayreuth is adopting the valuable device of tape-recording a performance and playing it back to the singers the next day. In principle it is rather like the French judicial method of confronting a murderer with the mangled body of his victim and watching his shudderings and blenchings. . . . (The singer) cannot ignore the evidence of his own ears. . . .'

other forms of microphone singing. The essential point is that, for physical reasons, singing on the half-voice into a microphone and obtaining volume by mechanical amplification does *not* result in the same timbre as singing with the full-voice without such amplification. However, it is possible to obtain good tone and to some extent save the voice, and in our opinion advantage should usually be taken of this mercy by busy singers.

There is, however, a class of singer who, by reason of a voice of small volume or some other limitation, is at pains to develop a microphone technique. Such a singer may be an artist and the result may be beautiful. But it is not to be regarded in the same way as singing in the concert hall or opera house; and artists of the latter are not advised to indulge in such practices at the same time. One technique may interfere with the other.

The reader will probably have had the melancholy experience of attending a concert to hear a singer he has admired on the radio or in films only to be greatly disappointed in the quality and power of the same voice without amplification. The moral to be drawn by singers should be obvious.

On the other hand some singers must modify intensity at certain pitches and timbres to avoid microphone distortion.

Modern uses of the microphone by 'pop-singers' and others will not be discussed here, but we have seen vocal damage in all these types of performer, as one would expect.

5

Why Voices 'Break Down';
Prevention and Treatment

Not unnaturally a professional voice user generally refrains from consulting a laryngologist until he suspects that there is something wrong with his throat. His symptoms usually fall under two heads: inability to sing or speak as well as he has been able to in the past, and sensations of discomfort referable to the throat. He is usually thinking more in terms of damage to the throat due to some form of *disease*,* than of laryngeal injury caused by *improper use* of the vocal mechanism. Actually our observations, and those of others, show that though throat inflammations due to bacteria and viruses are common, conditions due wholly or partly to vocal abuse are also very common. Many doctors, not being particularly interested in professional voice users, are content to dismiss the subject of the common throat inflammations by saying merely, 'Rest the voice for a week or so and it will clear up on its own—it's hardly worth while treating it.' The first half of this opinion may be true, but, as any singer or actor knows, it is quite impossible for him to take a week off every time he gets a common cold or sore throat with laryngitis. No management could afford to engage such an artist. So he works as long as he possibly can, and treatment to minimize the severity and reduce the duration of such an illness is very much worth while. But singing with an inflamed larynx is liable to cause damage; our policy, therefore, is always to keep such an artist at work *short of* risking any permanent or

* The word 'disease' is not to be understood as necessarily implying a dangerous or serious condition—the mildest 'common cold' or sore throat is medically speaking a disease. The term 'acute' means of relatively sudden onset and short duration; 'chronic' implies gradual onset and longer duration; these terms do *not* refer, as many laymen seem to think, to the *severity* of the illness.

serious damage, and to advise how best to get through with the minimum of strain on the organs concerned.

The fact that it is only the occurrence of such an inflammation that has brought the professional voice user to see the laryngologist should not prevent inquiry into the general structure and mode of employment of his vocal mechanism, as described in the two preceding chapters. Indeed we consider it an essential preliminary to giving well-founded advice and treatment based on a full and comprehensive diagnosis. We shall therefore in this chapter consider first conditions due to vocal abuse, and then those due to common inflammatory diseases.

It will, however, be appreciated that some repetition and overlapping is unavoidable—both of diseases with vocal abuse, and of one chapter's subject-matter with another's. We repeat that such repetition may not be a bad thing, and should at least emphasize the interdependence of the various aspects of the subject.

We advise and treat individual people, each with a particular personality, life history, mentality, body, habits and illness—not merely damaged organs or cases of text-book diseases. In addition it is an axiom of medical practice that history, symptoms and examination findings must be correlated and a *diagnosis* established. Treatment must then be directed, where possible, to *curing the disease*. Only then may measures be prescribed solely to *relieve symptoms* which are manifestations of this disease. This is where the lay public, encouraged by patent medicine advertisements, so often get the wrong idea. One receives requests for something to relieve a headache, sore throat, stuffy nose, etc., rather than for advice as to the discovery and eradication of the causative disease or dysfunction.

The *symptoms* of most of these conditions, as far as the throat is concerned, usually consist of some discomfort (aching, tightness, soreness, dryness, etc.) and of some impairment of vocal range and quality. Commonly there is difficulty in singing high notes *softly*, the reason being that thickened or irregular vocal cords or those with weakness of their muscle components cannot be stiffened and thinned, and so high notes can only be achieved by raising breath pressure and forcing air through tightly opposed cords—which notes cannot but be loud, as well as shrill (cf. Chap. 2). In other cases the singer complains that he has difficulty with his middle range of notes, the reason probably being that resort to the above method in some degree achieves the high notes, but when breath pressure is reduced and cordal opposing force lessened the thickened or muscularly weak cords can only vibrate at the slower rates resulting in low notes.

Conditions commonly encountered will now be described. Those interested enough to require more detailed accounts are referred to various papers by the author (Punt[66, 71]).

CONDITIONS DUE MAINLY TO
IMPROPER OR EXCESSIVE USE OF
THE VOICE

1. **Myasthenia of the Larynx (Phonasthenia).** It is largely the action of the muscles powering the vocal cords that brings about the constantly changing stiffness and thickness of their substance on which the pitch of the notes produced partly depends. Other muscles attached to various mobile parts of the jointed laryngeal framework also vary the cordal stiffness and position. Overwork of these groups of muscles causes them to tire, much the same as leg muscles tire after a long walk or bicycle ride. Inflammation of these muscles (myositis), such as may occur during an infective laryngitis, also weakens them. As a result the singer finds his voice becomes unreliable, and there is difficulty in achieving or sustaining particular notes. The muscles are acting most powerfully during sopranos' and tenors' high notes and these notes in such singers are therefore most often and most seriously affected.

Some degree of myasthenia usually accompanies all the conditions mentioned in this section, as well as cases of infective laryngitis. Diagnosis of the particular muscle-groups most severely involved, and of the relative importance of myasthenia in a singer also suffering from one of these other conditions, is a skilled procedure.

Myasthenia of the larynx is seen in many forms; one form tends to merge into another, but for convenience of reference they may be tabulated:

(a) *Acute*
    (*i*) Due to a brief period of severe vocal abuse. This may

be associated with acute engorgement of the blood vessels in the cords, and one or two may even rupture causing hæmatoma formation (bruising).

(*ii*) Due to myositis secondary to an infective laryngitis.

(b) *Subacute*

(*i*) Due to weeks or months of excessive or improper vocal use, whether professional, social or domestic.

(*ii*) In association with vocal nodules or other laryngeal condition.

(*iii*) In association with overwork, coughing from any cause, or any debilitating disease, including pulmonary tuberculosis.

(*iv*) On resumption of singing after a few weeks' holiday, such cases being comparable to beginning of season difficulties in athletics, before the muscular system gets back into training.

(*v*) Due to endocrine factors, such as menstruation and the menopause.

(*vi*) Due to emotional causes, especially if accompanied by much weeping.

(c) *Chronic*

(*i*) As for subacute, but continuing for years.

(*ii*) Senile. As elsewhere in the body the laryngeal muscles deteriorate with advancing years, but especially if they have been ill-used. There is also a reduction in intrinsic laryngeal reflexogenic systems. (Wyke[33, 34]). This is the condition that usually determines the age of a singer's retirement.

It is a matter for wonder that when a diagnosis of vocal myasthenia has been made and its cause explained, the artist often expresses surprise, even if he has been persuaded to admit to gross vocal overuse and abuse. It may be necessary to emphasize time and again that his profession involves vocal athletics, and that his laryngeal muscles deserve the same degree of care and consideration as is employed by the wise trainer of sportsmen or racehorses. If the performer could only visualize the amount of work he is asking his larynx to withstand, he would be amazed not at its eventual failure, but at its powers of endurance. It is hardly facetious to say that most artists need three larynges—one for professional purposes, one for social and domestic use, and a spare!

From the above, prevention and treatment should be fairly obvious and may be briefly grouped as follows:

(*a*) Vocal *rest* (not more exercise, by anybody's 'method to strengthen the voice' although the voice therapist will be valuable later).

In acute cases twenty-four hours' absolute silence is very strongly advised—and we know what an ordeal this is.

In subacute cases one to eight weeks of severely restricted vocal use may be necessary. We frequently advise the performer, during this period, never to speak an inessential word unless he is paid for it!

Beginning of season difficulties, however, should resolve if singing is resumed *gradually.*

In chronic cases the voice will probably have to be saved for occasional appearances.

(*b*) Treat the underlying cause or associated condition and learn to avoid vocal abuse.

(*c*) Certain substances, given systemically, may benefit muscles (their use has been publicised in regard to athletes and race-horses). These steroids are often extremely effective in improving singers' vocal performance; but considerable judgement and experience is needed; as they are particularly popular in U.S.A. one could say 'mandatory'!

(*d*) Factors involved in maturing and ageing of the voice have been considered in the previous chapter.

Obviously the prognosis varies enormously and no general guide can be given. Most acute and subacute cases recover if the artist and teacher are intelligent enough to face the facts when they have been explained, and will co-operate in treatment and management. Those who will not believe what they are told and persist in vocal abuse will eventually ruin their voices. Most singers are as old as their larynges, and although we are always hearing tales of sixty-year-old singers whose voices are still splendid, we more often meet those in their thirties, or even twenties, whose vocal powers are already ageing.

But in true senile mysathenia, which is often accompanied by an atrophy of the cordal covering, the singer should be gently but firmly advised that her career is drawing to a close. The wise artist, if financial considerations permit, will prefer to end her professional career with dignity, albeit sorrowfully, rather than continue a losing fight until all beauty has left her once-admired tones. Finance, the strange compelling influence of the stage and the importunity of impresarios or the public all tend to persuade the artist to continue long after her more discerning admirers would prefer only to remember her at her prime. A compromise may sometimes be achieved by restricting appearances to very occasional performances of those parts of her repertoire she can still perform with beauty.

Pressman and Keleman[26] state very factually that 'the larynx in senescence reflects the process of atrophy found elsewhere in muscles and mucosa with atrophic thinning, dehydration of the mucosa, loss of elastic tissues, and general atrophy of the muscles of the vocal cords themselves. . . . There are many individual differences but generally at 70 a true decline is inevitable.'

The author can confirm this, and is often saddened by these consultations.

'No man (voice) at all can be living for ever, and we must be satisfied'.

2. **Vocal Nodules of Attrition.** The normal vocal cords have smooth surfaces and no irregularities of their free borders. In the above condition there exists a nodule on the edge of each cord. The nodule on one cord is opposite to that on the other, and they arise at about the middle of the membranous cords— that is midway between the front end of the cord and the tip of the cartilage contained within its rear portion. Uncommonly only one cord may show a node, but we believe that in such a case the other cord will also develop one very shortly if steps are not taken to prevent it. Indeed, we have seen this happen.

During phonation this is just the region where the vibrating cords might be expected to strike most forcibly against one another, especially if the glottic shock method of attacking high notes is employed. The behaviour, occurrence and microscopic appearance of removed vocal nodules tend to support this method of production. They are commonest in sopranos and especially in those who have been shocking the glottis and forcing high notes. In fact the more sopranos' larynges one examines and the closer one looks at them, the commoner they seem to be—though frequently the irregularities are so minute as to cause little trouble. They are probably next commonest in mezzo-sopranos and tenors. They are also frequent in schoolmistresses, in mothers who shout at their children, in those with deaf relatives, in workers in noisy occupations and in poorly trained actors, especially those who have become used to working with a microphone and then endeavour to play a heavy part in the Theatre. They also occur in screaming or shouting children and are sadly common in child vocalists. Vocal abuse is always the cause. There exists a very beautiful ciné film of the phonating larynx of a young lady who becomes a cheer-leader to an American University team. By taking a few frames several times a week for some months, and then running the collection together, the photographer was able to show the nodules forming and enlarging.

Microscopic examination of removed nodules shows thickening of the membrane covering the cords, which progresses from soft swelling in recent examples (often with evidence of haemorrhage from damaged blood vessels) to hard, corny proliferations in long-standing specimens. The author has a series of histological colour transparencies of nodules he has removed which show these changes very clearly, and correlate well with the patients' vocal histories.

Two factors are, rather seldom, of significance in the production of acute haemorrhagic nodules: some people are particularly affected by aspirin, which may increase the tendency to haemorrhage as a response to trauma. Some female singers must not sing during menstruation, as in their case the vocal cords become oedematous at these times and engorged blood vessels may rupture. Medicinal treatment may prevent this, but the clause sometimes inserted into contracts which releases the singer from performance on certain days of the month is often a sensible precaution.

The symptoms resulting from vocal nodules are variable, and are usually complicated by the additional presence of myasthenia (weakness) of the laryngeal muscles which has also resulted from excessively forceful methods of vocalization—which are often perpetuated as the performer endeavours to overcome the mechanical handicap of the nodules. In well-marked cases the nodules interfere with the thinning and stiffening of the vibrating cords and thus affect the resulting tone. In some cases the main difficulty is with high notes (especially pianissimos or diminuendos), the singer having to use more and more effort, thereby forcing the cords more and more violently together, and thus inflicting increasing damage. In other cases the singer will declare she can still reach her high notes (which admission suggests she always has forced them) but finds the reduced breath pressure employed for her middle range of notes allows the nodules to sink slightly downwards where they are more directly in the glottic chink and impart a hoarse character to the tone. Eventually any endeavour to use the voice beyond a very limited range results in the note 'cracking'.

As with all the conditions mentioned in this section, prevention is better than cure. When vocal nodules have been diagnosed, however, it is essential to make the patient realize that their cause is vocal abuse and that as soon as possible treatment must *begin* with vocal rest (not more exercises by anyone's 'method to restore the voice'). The amount of rest necessary varies greatly from case to case, but success can often be achieved if the performer will reserve three weeks free from all engagements, keeping at first entirely silent (avoiding, especially, forced whispering) and then resuming gentle speech in quiet surroundings. Treatment is then largely in the hands of the patient and a careful teacher; singing or dramatic speaking should be resumed gradually and gently, and with no hurry to extend range or volume. When the performer can be trusted no longer to shock the glottis, even when the watchful teacher is not present, public appearances may be resumed, if possible in less-exacting rôles, as the nervous strain involved is considerable, and in addition the laryngeal muscles will fail if they are too suddenly reintroduced to arduous work. (Singing involves vocal athletics, and if an athlete has a period of rest, he returns to training gradually.) By this time examination will usually reveal that the nodules are smaller, or may even have disappeared, and that the texture of the cordal surfaces and condition of the laryngeal muscles have improved.

Sprays and other local applications to the larynx may be of help in enabling the player to carry on for a few days whilst arrangements are made for the rest period, but she must be made to understand the position, and prevented from pinning her faith on a throat spray to the neglect of the essential vocal rest and re-education. With some patients this is difficult!

In certain cases of persistent nodules, it is necessary to remove them with fine forceps introduced through an illuminated tube via the mouth, under a general anaesthetic. The operation is delicate, the responsibility considerable, and vocal rest as described above must follow. This operation has been greatly facilitated by the technique introduced by Kleinsasser, which involves the use of a brightly-illuminated operating microscopy, very fine instruments, and an anaesthetic technique allowing the surgeon plenty of time. However, the above considerations still apply.

The prognosis in vocal nodules varies greatly from patient to patient and depends to some extent on the condition of the laryngeal muscles. It is good with early nodes in co-operative performers, and bad in those who persist in vocal abuse. Minute nodules showing no tendency to increase in size as the years pass, as are often seen in experienced performers, are of less serious import, especially if the player is able to confine himself to easier vocal rôles in the future.

Finally, it is always worth considering whether the alleged soprano or tenor voice is not in fact better suited for the mezzo-soprano or light baritone range.

For further reading the enquirer is referred to the excellent books by Greene[58] and by Moore[63].

3. **Chronic Non-infective Laryngitis.** Although this common condition is generally seen in those who use their voice excessively, too loudly and with a forceful or harsh mode of production, these are not the only causative factors. Excessive smoking and spirit drinking are often indulged in, and there may be some truth in the contention of earlier laryngologists that there is an association with gout or some form of 'rheumatism'. We suspect that it would be more accurate to describe

this condition as a *diathesis*—a constitutional predisposition. Trouble begins most often in middle age, and the sufferers are usually male—although it is sad to record that there are plenty of husky actresses about and some are young in years, although their throats and voices exhibit vocal abuse dating from childhood. These chronic croakers tend to conform to a type—that of the sociable, garrulous, heavy drinking and smoking, often plethoric, individual conspicuously in evidence in any busy London pub, some of which friendly houses of entertainment are strategically situated in relation to stage-doors! Stuffy, dry, dusty, overheated atmospheres—particularly certain theatre dressing-rooms—make these throats worse. All the factors mentioned are generally present to some extent, and the resulting hoarseness is so characteristic that it is by tradition associated with the comic-paper's or music-hall artist's representation of newsvendors, publicans, bookmakers and sergeant-majors. It has also been named 'the gin and midnight voice'! In practice one meets with it in varying degrees of severity in most trades and professions, but it is particularly important in actors.

The surface of the vocal cords is normally smooth, pearly, glistening and (by reflected light) white, or showing only a little pinkness from very slightly dilated blood vessels. In professional voice users some further increase in pinkness may be accepted as normal, or at least physiological. In a well-marked case of the condition under discussion dilation of blood vessels makes the cords appear dusky red, their surfaces slightly roughened and dulled, and their edges a little irregular. The difference in appearance might be compared to that between fine white or faintly rose-pink slipper-satin, and rather rubbed red velvet. In addition similar changes are to be seen in the mucous membrane covering the pharynx and larynx elsewhere, and there is usually an excess of rather sticky mucus. All degrees of the condition are met with from slight cordal congestion and roughening to the well-marked state described.

The seriousness of the resulting symptoms varies according to the extent of the changes and the purpose for which the voice is required. Some degree of hoarseness and lowering of pitch of the speaking voice is to be expected as a result of the cordal thickening and roughening. Some actors are clever or fortunate enough to turn this to good account, the voice losing its purity and clarity but gaining a characteristic rich huskiness which can be rather attractive. The effect in a baritone may be similar as long as the changes are not very marked, when an unpleasant harsh or throaty tone results. In tenors, however, the consequence is much more serious, the purity of high notes being spoilt. The more the tenor (or light baritone) has been noted for the lyric, rather than for the dramatic, quality of his tone, the more serious is the effect. Women are less commonly affected, and fortunately so, for sopranos' and mezzo-sopranos' upper registers are particularly altered for the worse thereby and the actress, famous for her fascinatingly husky and sexy voice, will find in time that she is not quite so popular with managements and the public when the well-known tones are not only husky, but lacking in power, so that she cannot be heard and has to miss performances.

Prevention and treatment are difficult as little is known of the underlying predisposition of certain people to acquire the affection. Every effort must be made to reduce excessive consumption of alcohol and tobacco, and to minimize vocal abuse, but these patients are so often habituated to such indulgences, and to constant talking, that they find restrictions intolerable. As a compromise they may be persuaded to remain silent and abstinent for some hours before a performance and for an occasional complete day, with, to their ingenuous delight, considerable improvement in the voice. We have found in these cases occasional use of certain laryngeal spray solutions designed to diminish the (usually excessive) sensitivity of the larynx and to reduce the congestion of the mucosal vessels of great benefit, especially before a particularly important performance. These throats are usually dry and clogged with sticky mucus, and this can often be relieved. The very important question of lubrication of the larynx will be considered shortly. Many of these cases are of long-standing and a complete and permanent cure is not to be expected. Worsening of the condition should be regarded as an indication for *vocal rest*. If such worsening occurs just before an especially important performance it is often possible by the means outlined above to restore the voice for the time being, but the performance, will tend to leave the voice hoarser than before and subsequent rest will be all the more necessary.

We have met cases where the throat condition was used as an excuse to avoid some uncongenial or inconvenient appearance—but this is rare; nor is the performer handled very sympathetically. Rather more often one is asked to support a request to miss one or two performances in order to be fresh for an engagement which would be artistically or financially more rewarding a few days later. This is only very occasionally justifiable. If an artist's voice can only just manage to get through six evenings and two matinées, he has no right to accept a Sunday engagement. From the time he leaves the theatre on Saturday night, until he arrives there again on Monday evening he should be *silent*. In the long run he will be the gainer, although he will not understand this at the time.

We must repeat that the condition of the vocal muscles, which are always overstrained in such cases, is usually more important than the state of the cordal covering membrane. The possessor of a powerful voice with less than perfect timbre can often find employment; but a weak voice in repeated danger of failing is useless, and no manager should engage such a liability.

4. **Lubrication Problems.** In a previous chapter it was explained that the vocal cords are lubricated mainly by minute glands situated above them, which should secrete thin mucus in adequate quantities. They are the 'oil-cans' of the larynx. A performer's cords vibrate several hundred times a second and it is no wonder that their preservation depends to a large extent on their being well-lubricated. Slow-motion films of a singer's larynx show this fine mucus being squirted on to the cords, which are thus vibrating in an oily-looking fluid. Unfortunately the various factors controlling these glands are not fully understood, although some, such as emotion and atmosphere, have been mentioned. Lubrication may be inefficient if the glands secrete too little mucus so that the larynx is too dry, or if the mucus is too thick and thus tends to clog the glottis. Singers and actors usually recognize this problem once it has been mentioned to them. Treatment can be difficult. Preparations containing an iodine compound may be effective, or the nerve supply to the mucous glands may be stimulated. Certain sprays

may be of great value, but few people can use a spray so that the medicament reaches as far as the larynx, and a single treatment by a laryngologist may only be effective for a matter of hours.

This problem of deficient lubrication is so common, so important and so often unappreciated in diagnosis, that the author recently devoted his allotted time at a recent meeting of actors' and singers' laryngologists to speaking solely on the subject:

'A speaking or singing voice may fail when there is nothing wrong with the structure of the pharynx or larynx, but only a defect in the essential *lubrication* of the mechanism—and especially of the vocal cords. When one considers these rapidly vibrating structures, it seems clear that they can only be expected to withstand such exercise if they are lubricated by an adequate amount of thin mucus, especially from glands in the laryngeal ventricles. It is also advantageous if the whole of the pharynx is well lubricated. This is self-evident if one listens to a speaker in excellent voice except for his having to pause at intervals to "clear his throat". It is also noted in the nervous orator with his ineffectual sips of water taken to relieve dryness.

Considering certain singers' throats over a period of years, I have often noted that those which are well lubricated survive longer. The same, surely, is true of any other piece of machinery. With this in mind, I invariably consider lubrication when examining the throat of a professional voice user.

Many conditions which result in lubrication defects will be familiar, but will be listed briefly for completeness.

They include emotional factors (particularly "stage-fright"), nose and sinus conditions, excessive smoking and drinking, the sicca syndrome, medicaments (such as "cold cures") which inhibit mucous and salivary secretion, and also poor air-conditioning. Tracheobronchial secretions may enter the larynx from below and impede lubrication.

We have all seen films of the phonating and singing larynx, and discussion has usually been concerned with cordal configuration and movements. I have been particularly interested to observe the jets of mucus squirted onto the cords by the ventricular glands. Surely the amount and consistency of this mucus is important, and how could the cordal epithelium survive without it? This natural lubricant should be adequate in quantity and thin in consistency. The patient will often complain of too much mucus, when actually the trouble is that there is *too little mucus and it is too thick.'*

It should be added that proprietary tablets alleged to 'dry up a cold' or 'catarrh' (A meaningless term) may have a disastrous drying effect on the throat, as may many antihistamines. We would again suggest the use of efficient humidifiers.

5. **Contact Ulcer and Pachydermia of the Larynx.** These rather rare conditions consist of ulceration of the posterior ends of the vocal cords (contact ulcer), or a proliferation of epithelium in the same area. They are both seen most frequently in Americans, of the hard-talking, low pitched, business-man type, and usually result from the 'hammer-and-anvil' action of the vocal processes of the cords striking together and inflicting mutual damage on covering epithelium and the deeper cartilage. The only reason for including the conditions here is that they may be encountered in husky 'tough guy' types of actors who use this method of speech. Treatment in well-developed cases is difficult and the prognosis bad—especially as they usually drink and smoke excessively and have a compulsive psychological need to express themselves in this manner. Rarely very minor examples are encountered in baritones who have been posing as basso-profundos. These cases may recover if they will listen to reason.

6. **Uncomfortable Sensations in the Throat.** People other than professional voice users are not normally aware of their throats. Such awareness is usual in singers and actors because their minds are so much occupied with the production of carefully gauged tones and because their throats are especially liable to the various occupational affections described above. The trained performer, however, who uses the voice correctly should not normally be markedly aware of throat sensations. Complaint is usually made of excessive mucus, dryness, desire to swallow or clear the throat, soreness or aching. Examination and questioning will frequently reveal one of the conditions mentioned in this chapter. A particular variety has been named

'clergyman's sore throat'. The psychological factors emphasized in Chapter I may be particularly important.

However, singing and dramatic speaking may properly be regarded as forms of vocal *athletics*, and it is no more surprising that the muscles and joints of a performer's larynx should ache than it is of equivalent structures in the legs of a ballet dancer, the elbow of a tennis-player or the shoulders of a golfer. These joint-and-muscle-aches can be treated. Steroids and 'anti-rheumatic' preparations may be valuable when properly used. Unhappily, by the time a performer presents with such symptoms the more delicate muscles within the larynx (which most unfortunately do not protest their ill-usage by much aching) have frequently been reduced to such a state of myasthenia (as previously described) that re-habilitation takes time.

COMMON UPPER RESPIRATORY
INFLAMMATIONS DUE TO BACTERIA
OR VIRUSES

Being diseases, rather than vocally produced injuries, the treatment of these infections is much more in the hands of the medical man, and they will therefore only be considered briefly in this volume.

1. **Chronic Infective Laryngitis.** This disease is mentioned first because of its apparent similarity to the non-infective laryngitis dealt with in the previous section. Our object in not describing both types under one heading is to emphasize that a definite conclusion must be arrived at in each case as to whether or not there is an infective element of any significance present. The decision is often difficult. The sites of such sepsis are most commonly the nose and adjacent sinuses, the tonsils, teeth and gums, and the chest.

Treatment is on the lines suggested, but includes, fundamentally, elimination of the responsible sepsis.

2. **The 'Common Cold'.** The symptoms of these infections are far too well known for description to be necessary. The subject has been confused by a host of old wives' tales and by the deceptively optimistic advertisements of patent medicine vendors.

The following facts should be remembered: 'Colds' are due to infection of the nose and throat by viruses, which are minute living organisms. Several different viruses have been identified at the time of writing and many others may await discovery, so we are really considering a group of upper respiratory virus infections which are similar, but not identical, in nature. No substance has been found which can be administered to humans and will destroy any of these viruses, render them inactive, or give protection against them. No so-called coldcure or preventative, of the many which have been tested under scientifically controlled conditions, has been found effective. The list includes vitamins, vaccines and antihistamines. At the present time Britain and the U.S.A. are being subjected to intensive advertising of various tablets alleged to dry up a cold, reduce nasal congestion and rid the sufferer of nasal and post-nasal mucus (which is presumably what is to be understood by the over-used and almost meaningless term 'catarrh'). These tablets should not be taken, and actors and singers must be especially careful to avoid them, as some preparations so dry up the mucous glands of the throat that lubrication is severely impaired, as has been mentioned in a previous section. If a patient has a nasal allergy, antihistamine or ephedrine-like drugs may be useful; and other decongestant or mucolytic preparations are often of value. But these should only be used on medical advice after careful examination and diagnosis.

These virus infections can only be escaped by those susceptible to them if all contact with other sufferers can be avoided, and under ordinary conditions of city life this is impracticable. For performers it is impossible. If 'colds' are about in a community the susceptible will be infected, possibly by someone in the incubation stage before symptoms are noted. Nor is it likely that attention to diet or clothing or protection from climatic conditions will make any difference. My only suggestion here is to avoid being too affectionate when meeting children.

Probably some of the symptoms experienced in the later stages of these infections, when the nasal discharge changes from watery to thick and yellow, and discomfort or cough referable to the pharynx and larynx become troublesome, are due to secondary invading bacteria, which may be sensitive to antibiotics. At this stage it may certainly be justifiable for the doctor to prescribe these, but skill and experience are necessary.

Various symptomatic treatments are available which may reduce nose or throat discomfort in the several stages of a virus infection, and most of these are well known. Everyone has his own pet remedy.

3. **Influenza.** Much of the above applies to this disease, which is an infection due to a well-recognized virus, having several types, and which is also resistant to drugs, although attempts at protection by vaccines have had a limited success.

Again symptoms need not be described here, except to state that the disease in different individuals and epidemics varies from a very mild one (often rather loosely called an 'influenzal cold') to a very severe and dangerous one with many complications.

Its peculiar characteristic is that it appears to weaken the body's resistance to other organisms. Frequently the influenza itself is not so severe, but tends to be followed by one of many possible secondary infections. In other cases some symptoms (muscular pains, sore throat, headache, general bodily weakness) will persist for weeks for no discernible cause.

In addition influenza is notorious for leaving its victim mentally depressed. Realization that this is a common sequela often enables the sufferer to bear this with fortitude. It may sometimes be banished by a short course of certain fairly harmless stimulant tablets. Convalescence may have to be longer than one might expect from the duration and severity of the original disease.

4. **Acute 'Sore Throat' or Tonsillitis.** This infection is often caused by one of the common bacteria, although frequently a virus is responsible. The pharynx and larynx are both affected to a varying extent. If tonsils are still present, the most marked feature will probably be a tonsillitis. In addition the lymph glands at the side of the neck will be inflamed, as lymph vessels enter them from the throat. The larynx may almost escape infection or may be so severely inflamed as to render the patient nearly voiceless, the cords being a brilliant red and the underlying muscles also acutely inflamed. In some cases the upper

surface of the cords and larynx appear little affected, but the lower surface of the cords and trachea are inflamed. This and an accompanying myositis may render the patient much more hoarse than one would expect from laryngoscopic appearances. Pain is referred to the inflamed areas and there may be cough with, later, sputum. Swallowing, talking and traction or pressure on the neck may be painful. The patient feels ill and there is often fever.

When the infection is bacterial, a course of penicillin is usually the most effective cure, and for the most reliable and rapid response this is best given initially by intramuscular injection.

Relapse is not uncommon—possibly on account of the inaccesibility of organisms within the depths of the crypts with which the tonsils are pitted. Recurrences may be frequent due to the same cause or to re-infection.

Numerous preparations are available to relieve the various distressing symptoms. Aspirin is still one of the best pain relievers. Hot gargles of bicarbonate of soda solution and external application of heat to the neck may help and, if the glands are tender, immobilizing the neck in many layers of wool. Cough may be suppressed if there is no sputum, or made easier when sputum is present. In some cases mildly anæsthetic or decongestive throat sprays may be allowed. Steam inhalations, with or without medication, may be comforting. A hot bath in a hot room full of steam may be best of all. Copious fluids should be taken.

If the larynx is markedly involved the patient **must not** sing or act. Here it is that the laryngologist must stand firm in his refusal to agree to a performance. Disobedience may entail weeks or months away from the stage and has been known to ruin a larynx permanently. Absolute silence, that the acutely inflamed larynx may be at complete rest, is the ideal.

The above account is of a severe case. The infection may be of all degrees of severity and is usually much milder, calling for correspondingly less drastic measures. Careful judgment may be called for in borderline cases of to 'sing or not to sing'? or 'penicillin therapy or not'?

This is a suitable place to say something very briefly of the indications for removal of tonsils and adenoids. Speaking generally it is agreed that adenoids should be removed if they are obstructing either the nasal airways or the Eustachian tubes leading from the back of the nose to the middle ears. This state of affairs is common in childhood but rare after puberty. Properly performed the operation does no harm and its benefits, including those to vocal quality, may be considerable. Tonsils should be removed if there is a history of repeated attacks of tonsillitis. Occasionally young singers present with tonsils protruding far into the cavity of the throat, and in such cases their removal may improve the voice. Although it may take the singer a little while to get back into practice after a tonsillectomy, we have never known of a case where this operation, carefully performed for adequate reasons, has resulted in vocal impairment. Frequently the player is pleased to find even more benefit than was predicted from the operation. But the decision to advise tonsillectomy must be carefully considered, and one must resist any temptation to operate on an unsuccessful singer in the vague hope that the voice may be improved.

CANCER AND TUBERCULOSIS OF THE LARYNX

Most laryngeal conditions involve no danger to life and but little to bodily health. The above are exceptions and certain facts about them should be widely known.

1. **Cancer of the larynx** in many cases *if diagnosed early enough* can be cured without a painful or mutilating procedure. It is the extensive, late cases which lead to distressing death. A few weeks may make all the difference between these two alternatives. If everyone having *any* change in their speech persisting longer than a month were to be examined forthwith by a laryngologist, the majority of these cancers would be cured. There is no other *early* symptom; pain especially is usually late. The chances of any particular patient reporting with vocal symptoms having cancer are not great, and if nothing serious is found the relief to the patient's mind is enormous. Many patients fearing they may have cancer avoid the doctor,

dreading his diagnosis, until too late. By this procrastination they often needlessly sign their own death warrants.

2. **Tuberculosis of the larynx** is secondary to tuberculosis of the lungs. Occasionally weakness or hoarseness of voice may be the first symptom which leads to detection of the disease. The prognosis is that of the chest condition, but the laryngeal disease is usually healed by the action of anti-tuberculous drugs. As with cancer, early diagnosis is important and depends on the patient seeking medical advice promptly.

Benign tumours, cysts and polypi also arise occasionally in the larynx and may interfere with the vibration of the cords. Careful instrumental removal through the mouth is necessary. The prognosis as to voice is variable.

OTHER MATTERS AFFECTING THE HEALTH AND EFFICIENCY OF THE PROFESSIONAL VOICE USER

Among the common conditions *outside* the pharynx and larynx which may directly or indirectly affect the voice are diseases of the *nose* and related *sinuses* (particularly infections and allergic conditions), *ear* diseases (because of interference with hearing), *gynæcological* conditions, *chest* diseases (sometimes by involvement of the nerve supply to the laryngeal muscles), and *anæmia*, often due to bleeding hæmorrhoids or to excessive monthly loss in women. Any symptoms referable to these organs should be reported to the physician by a wise singer. Vitamins are fashionable, and correction of deficient intake is essential; but in spite of the advertisements vitamin deficiency today in Britain is rare, except in those taking very poor meals such as food cranks and certain elderly people living alone.

Some *hormonal* disturbances have already been mentioned, including the individually unpredictable changes of puberty. During menstruation the vocal cords may become swollen and increasingly vascular with a tendency to haemorrhage; some singers must not perform at these times. The contraceptive pill may be dangerous in young girls, causing the developing larynx to enlarge, lowering the tessitura and ruining sopranos' higher notes. Similar effects have been noted, also in young females, due to anabolic steroids, which, properly used, are valuable in restoring muscles weakened by a previous illness or overwork. These latter changes are permanent. The menopause may also contribute to vocal deterioration. Thyroid dysfunction occasionally needs consideration. (See Brodnitz[11] and also Pressman and Keleman).[26] Medical advice is necessary in all these problems.

Constipation is an evil, but abuse of purgatives is a commoner one. Again a physician's advice, and not advertisements', should be taken.

Finally, every man is a fool or a physician at forty. In other words avoid indulgences you have found by experience to disagree with you. Avoid rush, but obtain sufficient steady exercise and fresh air. Plan your day so as not to have expended the best of your vitality when the time of performance arrives. As age advances save yourself and your voice more and more for the performance, but especially the voice, which, alas, usually fails some years before the body.

6

Producers, Directors and Voices

Laryngologists who specialize in singers' and actors' vocal problems are accustomed to a pattern which occurs time and again during the familiar sequence of auditions, rehearsals, tour, pre-views, opening-performance and eventual 'run'—if any. Reading advance publicity in theatrical journals, and knowing most of the leading artists and their vocal capabilities, we can often forecast their troubles in advance and anticipate the expected panic telephone call within a day or two of its reception.

Many of these panic situations could be avoided if notice were taken of the advice given in this chapter—which 30 years of experience in the Theatre tells one is extremely unlikely!

It must be added that although the artist may be in some part to blame for his vocal trouble, it is seldom entirely his own fault; and although anxiety before a dreaded first-night is often contributory, such cases are never 'all nerves', as some managements like to believe.

The various factors frequently responsible for threatened disasters will now be described:

1. It is unwise to engage a much-publicised 'Star' to play a part without considering whether the voice is capable of sustaining the role. This applies particularly to film or television personalities, many of whom are unable to perform efficiently without a microphone and a studio sound-system.

2. Singing, acting and dancing are all different arts, requiring different training and disciplines. Few performers excel in more than one activity. Your fine actor is unlikely to be able to cope with the vocal demands of a 'big musical', and your dancer even less-likely. Yet one meets such really absurd problems every week. It is nothing unusual to greet an elegant, long-legged lady declared as a singer, to ask her when she gave up dancing, and to be answered, 'a few weeks ago, when I got this part'. She will acknowledge that it took her many years to learn to dance, but she and her management seem surprised that she cannot be expected to learn to sing during a 6-week period of rehearsals!

3. Successful performers are much in demand and **'avail-ability'** is often a problem. A sensible Management will secure *sole* rights to a performer's services, permitting no other engage-ments—not even for charity, or for advertising the production.

4. Rehearsals and Previews. It is the custom to work up to a crescendo of activity during final rehearsals and pre-views before the first-night. It makes no difference whether rehear-sals, tour, and pre-views have lasted six weeks or six months; there is always that last minute, shortage-of-time, overworked and lack-of-sleep, last-minute rush. Theatrical folk work that way for reasons of temperament. Admittedly they often achieve a fine First-Night, having worked themselves up to a high pitch of nervous energy. Nonetheless, it would often be better—and would certainly take better care of hard-worked voices—if the pace could be slowed down, instead of speeded-up, as the im-portant evening approaches. Although the idea will be regarded as revolutionary, and quite contrary to the way Man-agements and artists are accustomed to work, it is suggested that on the morning before the Opening day the entire Com-pany should be 'called', and the director should then dismiss them, putting them on their honour to spend the time relaxed and *quiet* until they arrived at the theatre the following evening.

5. With new musical productions the Management often want the **L.P. recording** on sale in the theatre by or before the first-night. This means yet more work for tired voices. We suggest that the 'sleeve' with order form and address-label would suf-fice, the actual recording being delayed for a week or two, when the voices will have had some rest.

6. All performers hate **mid-week matinées.** In many productions the box-office would lose nothing by doing away with them—to the voices' benefit.

7. Understudy rehearsals are commonly delayed until sometime after the opening performance. This is unwise, as 'cover' is most likely to be needed in the early weeks, when the principals' voices have not recovered from the production weeks.

8. Ideally an actor or singer should breathe **pure, clean, fresh well-humidified air.** In fact most dressing-rooms in Theatres and Opera Houses are hot, dry, dusty and dirty, the atmosphere being relieved here and there by an icy draught from an open door. More intelligent use of heating and ventilating systems, and particularly the installation of modern humidification equipment, would be of great benefit.

The much-travelled International Artist is particularly vulnerable in this respect, aircraft and hotel-rooms also being poorly air-conditioned. He should travel with a portable humidifier.

9. Performers, and their voices, need occasional **holidays**—and in the case of singers, a *gradual* return to vocal work. 'Agents', particularly, are slow to realize this—for obvious reasons.

10. The relationship between **singer, director and musical-director** may be very delicate. Some conductors are helpful and sympathetic to singers; others regard them merely as a nuisance, interfering with their 'musical interpretation'. (See Alexander[36]).

A long article could be written on this subject, but the essentials are simple:- if the orchestra is too loud for the singer's voice, make it quieter; if the tessitura is wrong for the singer (usually too high) either change the pitch or get another singer!

11. Lastly, a word about **lighting and acoustics.** An artist is more easily heard if there is some light on his face. Instead of leaving the lighting until very late in production, it would help if the main cues were set earlier. Some designers are so proud of themselves that they arrange for the lighting to be adjusted to show-off their scenery, leaving the performers in the dusk.

Acoustically voices sound of better quality in a well-filled auditorium than in an empty one. This fact should reassure a nervous novice rehearsing in a big theatre. The technical matter of the acoustics of theatres and concert-halls is far too complicated for discussion here, but at least Managements and performers could bear the matter in mind before committing themselves. We know one theatre which has been described by a percipient critic as 'the place where bad audiences go when they die'!

7
Fallacies and Traditions

SOCRATES. He who first gave names gave them according to his conception of the things which they signified, and if his conception was erroneous ... shall we not be deceived by him?
—PLATO. Cratylus.

The teacher of singing or voice production assumes great responsibility and may give enormous help or cause considerable harm.

The inquiring singer who reads books on the subject, attends several teachers and listens to advice from various colleagues finds it difficult to know whom to believe. The variety of views encountered increases the difficulty, especially as the singer is unlikely to have received training in scientific assessment of evidence, the critical approach to a problem or theory, or even in simple logic. The temptation to give detailed evidence in support of every statement and contention in this book has had to be resisted for reasons of space and for fear of confusing the reader, who, it is hoped, will at least realize that the account hangs together. The most we have been able to do is to indicate where statements are based on observations of our own, reports of others, fundamental facts and laws of anatomy, physiology and physics, or sound principles of pathology, therapeutics and clinical medicine. Unfortunately certain writers on singing who have a very scanty and muddled understanding of these subjects frequently claim that their methods have a scientific basis. It is as if a man with an imperfect knowledge of the multiplication table were to produce a mathematical theory. The main purpose of this final chapter, therefore, is to examine some of the commoner fallacies connected with singing, that the reader's mind may be cleared of a deal of rubbish and made more receptive and critical.

Perhaps the commonest retort of anyone whose methods of teaching or treatment have been questioned is: 'They *must* be sound, or how do you account for my successful results?' Critically minded and impartial observers know that this argument is fallacious and, in the case of singers' advisers, for the following reasons:

(*a*) If the potentialities of a singer's vocal equipment are good, teaching would have to be bad indeed to eliminate all beauty from the outset.

(*b*) The teacher may persuade herself, and by reason of her personality and prestige convince her pupil, that the latter's vocal mechanism is executing certain movements, and that the air stream and sound waves are behaving in certain ways, when in reality nothing of the sort is happening.

(*c*) Great singers and well-known teachers publish their theories and methods. They are all different! A day's reading in a public library will confirm this. A few examples are given in the bibliography. Note especially Shakespeare's[51] quotations from teachings of the 'old masters' of singing.

(*d*) The body tends to recover from many affections in time without treatment; the honest doctor knows that in most cases he is merely helping 'Dame Nature' to heal his patient, valuable though his help may be.

(*e*) Psychological reasons. In any bodily disease or dysfunction these play an important part in determining the patient's reaction as an individual to his affection. Confidence in his adviser, medical or otherwise, plus the reassurance that the latter is often able to give, is always a valuable part of his contribution. Unfortunately the charlatan knows this only too well; conversely the well-meant, but mistaken, adviser may be deluded into over-estimating the real value of his treatment or tuition.

Now follows consideration of certain popular fallacies of *vocal function*.

1. *Sung tones cannot be 'produced' or 'generated' in the pharynx or nose or head or anywhere except in the glottis, in the sense implied by most users of the phrase.*

Airborne sound means air thrown into rapid vibration, and it can only be set in vibration by another vibrating structure or structures. Though a column of air forced through a partly open glottis (as in whispering and in certain cases of cordal paralysis) and then through the pharynx and mouth can be set into vibration by means of the shape and consistency of the walls of those cavities, causing them to act as resonators and stops, such sounds are comparatively weak. Only the much greater vibrations set up by forcing air through nearly opposed cords are sufficient for ordinary speech or song. The functions of the pharynx and mouth are to act as resonators to augment and modify the essential larynx tones, and to form stops allowing of consonant formation.

Cranks arise from time to time who deny that the larynx is an organ of voice. One persevering gentleman has devoted years in an endeavour to show that tones are produced in the paranasal sinuses, undaunted by the fact that extensive surgery on those cavities or their becoming filled with pus or polypi or a radio-opaque solution has comparatively little effect on the voice. None of these theories is based on satisfactory evidence, and rather than waste space by refuting each in turn, we shall indicate the nature of the evidence proving that the larynx is, in fact, the source of voiced sounds:

(*a*) A vast amount of recorded observation by many laryngo-logists enables one to associate laryngeal lesions with vocal defects. No one whose profession entails daily observation of irregularities and tumours of various parts of the larynx, different types of interference with vocal cord movement and the effect of inflammations, and who consequently notes the influence of these conditions on vocal quality, could possibly doubt the vocal importance of the larynx.

(*b*) The account given in Chapter 2, supplemented by more detailed descriptions in works of anatomy, physiology and physics, hangs together so well that the basic mechanism by which human speech and song is produced can be readily understood. Though details of control of pitch and timbre are complex, description of fundamentals reveals no inconsistencies.

2. *So-called 'chest' and 'head' notes are not due to selective resonance in the chest and head*, nor in the paranasal air sinuses, nasal cavities or face ('the masque'). The work of Paget[24] and Russell[28] may be referred to.

Resonance from the chest cavity (probably the contained air tubes) may add richness to low notes; but this cannot be selective as it is not under the singer's control, except that the chest dimensions (and the tubes' diameters) lessen during expiration, and yet tone quality in a trained singer does not greatly vary according to the degree of inflation of the chest.

The nasal cavities and the cavities of the communicating sinuses are not as important as is generally believed. The teaching of Jean de Reszke, or possibly the misunderstanding or misreporting of the teaching, did a lot to focus overmuch attention on these cavities (see Stanley[52, 53]).

However, this is not necessarily to say that *sensations* of vibration or tingling in any region may not help a singer to produce a beautiful and unforced tone; but the error lies in wrongly attributing such sensations to physical phenomena such as resonance. Actually the sensations may be quite incidental and unconnected with the tone quality, which results from soundwaves arising elsewhere in the pharynx or mouth.

3. *Sound cannot be 'thrown' or 'projected' and the palate or teeth cannot act as a 'sounding-board' to reflect sound waves from their surface*, though sound may be to some extent directed according to the direction in which the mouth is inclined, and the position, shape, inclination and consistency of these surfaces may modify the waves. Sound-waves are motion passed from particle to particle of air; the tracheal air itself only travels a few inches or feet. Sound-waves can only be reflected by a surface which is large in comparison to their wave-lengths. Paget[24] found that the range of basses' wavelengths being 3 to 14 ft. and sopranos' 1 to 4 ft., their palates would have to measure 20 sq. ft. and 6 sq. ft. respectively for them to reflect their sung tones!

4. *The 'Open Throat'*. Bartholomew[8] in an article entitled 'The

Paradox of Voice Teaching,' showed that for good tone and resonance the throat should be large, relaxed and low, not small, constricted and high. Bunch's[13, 14] researches on the "covered voice" confirm. Any instruction, imagery or sensation which helps the singer to attain this is therefore valuable, and he includes under this heading such terms as 'opening the throat,' 'singing in the masque,' etc. In other words, such terms do not mean anything scientifically, but may help the student to do the right thing.

5. *Manipulations and exercises of certain structures of the neck, larynx, throat and tongue in an endeavour to strengthen certain muscle groups.* Though part of the stock in trade of most singing teachers and elocutionists, we find it difficult to believe that many of these vocal gymnastic exercises and manipulations really achieve their object. Certainly few of them are likely to strengthen muscles on physiological grounds (we do not refer to increasing control over them) and weakening of muscles through excessive vocal exercise is so common in singers as to be decidedly the more likely outcome. What most singers in search of strengthening exercises, like most patients in search of a tonic, really need, is *rest*.

As has already been stated, most singers and teachers who talk about 'diaphragmatic breathing' are really referring to control of abdominal wall muscles. The diaphragm becomes active during *inspiration* (Wyke).[33, 34]

6. *'Naturalness' of Song.* Many teachers make a virtue of what they like to regard as a 'natural' method of singing. This, as far as it is applied to a trained professional singer, is nonsense; her performance would be better described as vocal acrobatics, and is the result of long years of training enabling art to be superimposed on natural endowments—as in pianists, violinists, painters, or for that matter trick cyclists and jugglers, none of whose feats does one see performed elsewhere in nature. Negus[22, 23] in his masterly books on the evolution and comparative anatomy of the larynx, has shown that purposive production of sound as a means of communication is a very late use of the larynx, when one considers that organ throughout the animal kingdom. He also shows that it is the *mental* superiority of man, even more

than the anatomical suitability of his larynx, that has enabled him so vastly to exceed all other animals in expressing shades of meaning and in complexity of speech. In Chapter 3 we have tried to show wherein lie the additional factors rendering the fine singer different from the poor one.

Evolutionally the primary function of the larynx is to act as a valve keeping food and drink out of the lower air passages. Other important functions it has acquired include those in connection with respiration, olfaction, swallowing, cough (protecting the lower air passages from harmful secretions) and fixation of the chest wall. The latter action is very important in any muscular effort involving the upper limbs, the closed glottis preventing expulsion of air and so fixing the chest. To demonstrate this, try moving a heavy piece of furniture by pushing; try again during expiration through the mouth and note the much reduced available power of the upper limbs. This has some importance in singing, for such an action can take place immediately before attacking a note, and if it does, the action tending to oppose the cords may continue sufficiently long for them to strike one another whilst vibrating (the *coup de glotte*, see Chapter 4). Therefore do not when attacking a note adopt any such tendency to fix the chest, nor allow any forceful action or tension of the upper limbs.

Traditions and fallacies in connection with the *health of the throat* have been mentioned in the previous chapter, but we may conclude with one or two particular observations:

1. *Medicaments intended to improve the condition of the vocal cords.* Very many of these preparations have been used in the past, and one is always hearing of this or that miraculous remedy. The first important point is that no good may be expected unless the medicament is able to reach the desired site of action. As far as the larynx is concerned this rules out gargles. Substances such as penicillin, after absorption, can reach it via the blood stream, some volatile preparations can be applied by means of steam inhalations (soothing, but otherwise of doubtful value), but most medicaments are best delivered by a fine spray with a down-pointing tip (such as the de Vilbiss). By this method *decongestive*, *sedative* or *cleansing* solutions may be used

with benefit in suitable cases.

Astringents or so-called *stimulants* are of more doubtful value, and it is certain that the more caustic preparations, such as strong solutions of silver nitrate, often employed by laryngologists in the past, are very likely to do harm. The temptation always has been to over-treat the larynx and to over-value local applications. However, it is an interesting observation in psychology that patients more readily obey the injunction to remain silent for twenty-four hours 'because of the treatment just given to the cords', than if the latter is omitted. The greater part of the resulting benefit is likely to be derived from the vocal *rest*.

It must again be emphasized that diagnosis should proceed treatment, and that terminology should be as exact as possible. The word 'laryngitis' by itself means little, and may imply either infection or vocal abuse of various types. 'Catarrh' is a useless term, but the American 'post-nasal drip' is, at least, descriptive.

2. *Foods and Drinks.* Here we could make an entertaining collection of recipes handed down from generation to generation in husky tap-room confidences or hypochondriacal dinner-party anecdotes. They range from the horrid gargle with port and lemon, reminiscent of Mr. Silas Wegg[75] who gave his readings on gin and water as it 'mellers' the voice, to *Soup à la Cantatrice* made with cream and eggs, and the traditional stout and oysters. We believe that some of these delicacies are comforting to inflamed or irritable mucous membranes by reason of their demulcent properties. Milk, or warm drinks made with honey or syrup, for example, are soothing, and may allay cough. Alcohol, however, is more often harmful to the inflamed throat, although wines, beer and especially stout seldom do harm and the latter may be helpful. If we have been unduly critical of singers' and actors' cherished beliefs, let us end our book with that acknowledgement of a comforting tradition!

Bibliography

Publications have been classified according to the subjects for which they have been *mainly* consulted or referred to, in the case of those which could have been placed under more than one heading. Biographies, however, have been listed together.

The numbers below correspond to those appended to the authors' names in the text.

PHYSICS OF SOUND
1. Bartholomew, W. T. (1934). 'Physical Definition of "good voice quality" in the Male Voice.' *J. accoust. Soc. Amer.*, **6**, 25.
2. Fletcher, H. (1929). *Speech and Hearing*. Macmillan London.
3. —— (1934). 'Loudness, Pitch and the Timbre of Musical Tones and their relation to the Intensity, the Frequency and the Overtone Structure.' *J. accoust. Soc. Amer.*, **6**, 59.
4. Helmholtz, H. (1885). *The Sensations of Tone*. Trans. by A. J. Ellis. Longmans, Green, London.
5. Sundberg, J. (1977). 'The Acoustics of the Singing Voice.' *Scientific American.*, 236, **3**, 82.
6. Tyndall, J. (1883). *Sound*. 4th edit. Longmans, Green, London.
7. Wood, A. (1947). *The Physics of Music*. 4th edit. Methuen, London.

ANATOMY, PHYSIOLOGY AND EVOLUTION OF THE VOCAL MECHANISM
8. Bartholomew, W. T. (1940). 'Paradox of Voice Teaching'. *J. accoust. Soc. Amer.*, **9**, 446.
9. Bellussi, G. and Visendaz, A. (1949). 'Il problema dei registri vocati alla luce della roentgen-strati-grafica.' *Arch. ital. Otol.*, **60**, 130.
10. Brackett, I. P. (1948). 'Vibration of Vocal Folds at Selected Frequencies.' *Arch. Otolarying., Chicago.* **47**, 838.
11. Brodnitz, F. S. (1953). *Keep Your Voice Healthy*. Harper, New York.
12. Brodnitz, F. S. (1975). 'The Age of the Castrato Voice.' *J. Speech and Hearing Disorders*, **40**, 3.
13. Bunch, M. (1976). 'A Cephalometric Study of Structures of the Head and

93

Neck During Sustained Phonation of Covered and Open Qualities.' *Folia Phoniatrica*, **28**, 321.

14. Bunch, M. and Sonninen, A. (Oct. 1977). 'Some Further Observations on Covered and Open Voice Qualities.' *NATS Bulletin*, U.S.A.

15. Garcia, M. (1885). 'Observations on the Human Voice.' *Proc. roy. Soc.*, **7**, 399.

16. Gould, W. J. and Okamura, H. (1974). 'Respiratory Training of the Singer'. *Folio Phoniatrica*, **26**, 241.

17. Guthrie, D. (1938). 'Physiology of the Vocal Mechanism.' *Brit. med. J.*, **2**, 1189.

18. Hemery, H. (1939). *The Physiological Basis of the Art of Singing*. Lewis, London.

19. Hinchcliffe, R. and Harrison, D. Chap. 40 by Wyke, B. (1976). *Scientific Foundations of Otolaryngology*, W. Heinemann Medical Books, London.

20. Hollien, H. (1972). 'Vocal Registers'. *Fonoaudiologica*, Buenos Aires, **18**, 130.

21. Jackson, C. and Jackson, C. L. (1935). 'Dysphonia plicae ventricularis.' *Arch. Otolaryng., Chicago*, **21**, 157.

22. Negus, V. E. (1929). *The Mechanism of the Larynx*. Heinemann, London.

23. —— (1949). *The Comparative Anatomy and Physiology of the Larynx*. Heinemann, London.

24. Paget, R. A. S. (1930). *Human Speech*. Kegan Paul, London.

25. Pressman, J. J. (1942). 'Physiology of the Vocal Cords.' *Arch. Otolaryng., Chicago*, **35**, 355; and (1938). 'Action of the Larynx.' *Proc. R. Soc. Med.*, **31**, 1179.

26. Pressman, J. J. and Kelemen, G. (1955). 'Physiology of the Larynx'. *Physiological Reviews*, **35**, 506.

27. Punt, N. A. (1974). 'Lubrication of the Vocal Mechanism.' *Folia Phoniatrica*, **26**, 287.

28. Russell, G. O. (1931). *Speech and Voice*. Macmillan, New York.

29. Semon, F. (1892). 'The Culture of the Singing Voice.' *Not. Proc. roy. Instn.*, **13**, 317.

30. Various Authors (1949). 'High pitched Voice in Adult Male'. *Brit. med. J.*, **2**, 1246, 1426 and 1540.

31. Vennard, A. B. (1967). *Singing, the Mechanism and the Technique*, Carl Fischer, New York.

32. Von Leden, H. (1961). 'The Mechanism of Phonation.' *Auch. Otolaryng., Chicago*, **76**, 660.

33. Wyke, B. (1974). *Ventilatory and Phonatory Control Systems*. Oxford University Press, London.

34. Wyke, B. D. (1974). 'Laryngeal Myotactic Reflexes and Phonation.' *Folia Phoniatrica*, **26**, 249.

—— 'Laryngeal Neuromuscular Control Systems in Singing'. *ibid.*

VOICE TRAINING AND THEORIES
AND ÆSTHETICS OF SINGING

35. Aikin, W. A. (1900). *The Voice*. Macmillan, London.

—— (1910). *The Voice*. Longmans, Green, London.

36. Alexander, A. (1971). '*Operanatomy*' Orion. Messina. Italy.
37. Brown, O. L. (1975). Diagnostic Techniques for Evaluating Voice of Singer and Actor. *O.R.L. Digest.* **37**, 16.
38. Browne, L. and Behnke, E. (1st pub. 1883). *Voice, Song and Speech*, 23rd edit. Samson Low, London.
39. Cathcart, G. C. (1912). 'Voice Production.' *In* Latham and English. A System of Treatment. Churchill, London, **3**, 331.
40. —— (1951). 'Obituary of.' *Brit. med. J.*, **1**, 98.
41. Curtis, H. H. (1898). *Voice Building and Tone Placing.* Appleton, New York.
42. Field-Hyde, F. C. (1950). *The Art and Science of Voice Training.* Oxford University Press, London.
43. Froeschels, E. (1948). *Speech and Voice Correction.* Philosophical Library, New York.
44. Fucito, S. and Beyer, B. J. (1922). *Caruso and the Art of Singing.* Unwin, London.
45. Greene, H. Plunket. (1921). *Interpretation in Song.* Macmillan, London.
46. Guthrie, D., Milner, A., Paget, R., Curry, R. and Horsford, C. (1938). 'Discussion on Functional Disorders of the Voice.' *Proc. R. Soc. Med.*, **32**, 447.
47. Moses, P. J. (1948). 'Vocal Analysis.' *Arch. Otolaryng., Chicago*, **48**, 171.
48. Rumsey, H. St. J. (1950). 'Voice Strain.' *J. Laryng.*, **64**, 708.
49. Schatz, H. A. (1938). 'Art of Good Tone Production.' *Laryngoscope, St. Louis*, **48**, 656.
50. Seashore, C. E. (1919). *The Psychology of Musical Talent.* Silver, Burdet & Co., U.S.A.
51. Shakespeare, W. (1954). *Plain Words on Singing.* Putnam, London.
52. Stanley, D. (1935). *Your Voice.* Pitman, U.S.A.
53. —— (1948). *The Science of Voice.* Carl Fisher, New York.
54. Tetrazzini, L. (1923). *How to Sing.* Pearson, London.
55. Walshe, W. H. (1881). *Dramatic Singing.* Kegan Paul, London.

DISEASES AND DYSFUNCTIONS
56. Brodnitz, F. S. (1971). 'Hormones and the Human Voice.' *Bulletin of the New York Academy of Medicine*, **47**, 183.
57. Critchley, M. and Henson, R. A. *Music and the Brain.* Heinemann Medical Books Ltd., 1977.
58. Greene, M. C. L. (1964). '*The Voice and its Disorders.*' Pitman, London.
59. Jackson, C. and Jackson, C. L. (1937). *The Larynx and its Diseases.* Saunders, Philadelphia and London.
60. —— —— (1945). *Diseases of the Nose, Throat and Ear.* Saunders, Philadelphia and London.
61. James, I. M. *et al.* 1977. *Lancet. 8045.* 952.
62. Kleinsasser, O. (1968). *Microlaryngoscopy and Endolaryngeal Microsurgery.* Saunders, Philadelphia.
63. Moore, G. P. (1971). '*Organic Voice Disorders*'. Prentice-Hall, New Jersey.
64. Perello, J. (1954). *Clinica y Tratamiento de los Trastornos de la Voz de la Palabra.* M. Marin, Barcelona.
65. Phillipson, J. *Brit. Med. J.* 1978. *6121.* 1209.

66. Punt, N. A. (1968). 'Applied Laryngology—Singers and Actors'. *Proc. Roy. Soc. Med.* **61,** 1152.
67. —— (1969). 'Vocal Disabilities of Singers and Actors'. *The Practitioner,* **202,** 650.
68. —— (1973). 'Treatment of Singers' and Actors' Throats.' *Excerpta Medica.* **337,** 602.
69. —— (1973). 'Management of E.N.T. Disabilities of Singers'. *Proc. Roy. Soc. Med.* **66,** 1073.
70. —— (1975). 'Diagnostic Techniques for Evaluating Voice of Singers and Actors: Problems of Stress'. *O.R.L. Digest.* **37,** 6.
71. Punt, N. A. World Medicine. 1977 *12.* 24.

BIOGRAPHIES AND MISCELLANEOUS

72. Agate, J. (1946). *A Shorter Ego.* Vol. 2. Harrap, London.
73. Bolitho, H. (1936). *Marie Tempest.* Sanderson, London.
74. Caruso, D. (1945). *Enrico Caruso.* Simon and Schuster, New York.
75. Dickens, C. (1864–5). *Our Mutual Friend.* Chapman and Hall, London.
76. Edwardes, T. (1946). *The Lore of the Honey-Bee.* 19th edit. Methuen, London.
77. Lehmann, L. (1938). *Wings of Song.* Trans. by M. Ludwig. Kegan Paul, London.
78. Tauber, D. N. (1949). *Richard Tauber.* Art and Education. London.
79. Terry, E. (1908). *The Story of My Life.* Hutchinson, London.
80. Whyte, F. (1898). *Actors of the Century.* Bell, London.

Index

ACOUSTICS, 84–85
Actors, characteristics of, 1
Adenoids, removal of, 79
Æolian tones, 31
Agate, James, 11
Alcohol, 10, 11, 59, 71, 92
   see also Drinking
Amplification, 60
Anaemia, 80
Anatomy, knowledge of, 14–15
Antibiotics, 76
Antihistamines, 74, 76
Anxiety, 3, 5, 6, 9, 11, 40, 82
Articulation, 27, 46, 58
Artistic temperament, 2
Aspirin, 78
Astringents, 92
Atmospheric conditions, 59, 84
Availability, 83

BARRISTERS, 13
Bartholomew, W. T., 37, 51, 89
Bellows. See Lungs
Bernouille effect, 31
Beta-blocker, 10
Blood vessels, dilation of, 70
Bone-conduction, 36
Breath control, 45
Breathing
   diaphragmatic, 90
   without constriction or dis-
      comfort, 57
Broadcasting, 59
Bronchi, 36
Bronchial tubes, 21
Brown, Oren, 43, 51, 58

CANCER of larynx, 79
Cannabis, 10

Cantors, 12
Caruso, Enrico, 4, 46
Castration, 56
Catarrh, 76, 92
Cathcart, G. C., 52
Chaliapin, 46
Character, 47
Chest cavity, 21, 89
Chest diseases, 80
Chest notes, 89
Chest requirements, 41
Chest resonance, 36
Children's voices, 54
Choristers, 12
Cilia, 21
Clergy, 12
'Clergyman's sore throat', 12, 75
Clowns, 3
Cold cures, 76
Common cold, 75–77
Confidence, 4
Consonants, 16, 35
Constipation, 81
Contact ulcer, 74
Contraceptive pill, 80
Coup de glotte, 50, 90
Covered voice, 29, 90
Crico-thyroid muscle, 23, 33
Cysts, 80

DECONGESTANTS, 76
Depression, 3
de Reszke, Jean, 89
Diathesis, 70
Directors, advice for, 82
Doctor-patient relationship, 7
Drinking, 69, 70, 73, 92
   see also Alcohol
Drugs, 9–12

Dry throat, 11, 71, 74, 76

EAR diseases, 80
Edge tones, 31
Edwardes, Tickner, 14
Emotional factors, 2, 73
Emotional stress, 8
Epiglottis, 31
Exercises, muscular, 90
Expiration, 17
Extravagance of actors, 2

FALLACIES, 86–92
False cords, 31
'Falsetto tenors', 56
Field-Hyde, F. C., 42, 59
First-nights, 4, 82, 83
Flexibility, 46
Food recommendations, 92
Frequency of singing, 56
Fucito, S., 43
Fundamental pitch, 25

GARGLES, 91
Glottic shock, 50, 66
Glottis, 88
  anatomy, 17
  timing of the opening, closing and
    shut phases of, 31
Gout, 69
Greene, H. Plunket, 15, 58
Gynaecological conditions, 80

HARMONICS, 18, 31, 38
Hazlitt, William, 2
Head notes, 89
Health and stamina requirements,
  41
Hearing, examination, 41
Heart-rate, 10
Helmholtz, H., 34
Hoarseness, 70, 71, 80
Holidays, 84
Hormonal disturbances, 80
Huskiness, 70, 71

INFLUENZA, 77
Inspiration, 17, 90

Intelligence, 47
Intensity, 16, 22, 25, 26, 30, 44
Irving, Henry, 5

JACKSON, C. and C. L., 53, 56

KEITH, Sir Arthur, 14
Keleman, G., 66

LAMPERTI, 54
Laryngeal mucus, 41
Laryngeal spray, 71
Laryngitis
  chronic infective, 75
  chronic non-infective, 69
  infective, 63
Larynx, 26
  anatomy, 17
  cancer of, 79
  damage to, 52
  examination, 6, 41
  function of, 33
  health of, 5
  in senescence, 66
  inflamed, 61, 78
  myasthenia of, 56, 63–66, 68
  overworking muscles of, 52
  pachydermia of, 74
  primary function of, 91
  requirements for fine singing,
    33–34
  tuberculosis of, 80
  vocal importance of, 88
Lecturers, 12
Lehmann, Lotte, 49
Leisure, 7
Lighting, 84
Loudness, 30, 56
Lubrication, 11, 21, 72–74
  conditions impeding, 73
  deficient, 72–73
Lungs
  anatomy, 16
  as bellows, 16
    requirements for fine singing, 32

MANAGEMENT, 83
Matinées, 84

Melba, Dame Nellie, 14
Membranes, 21
Menopause, 81
Menstruation, 80
Mental attitude, 1
Microphone, 60, 67
Moses, P. J., 42
Mouth, 38
  examination, 41
  resonance, 35
  resonating cavities, 18–20
  role of, 16
Muscle weakness, 56
Muscular aching, 52, 75
Muscular action, 11
Muscular contraction, 51
Muscular exercises, 90
Musical appreciation, 55
Musical interpretation, 84
Myasthenia of larynx, 56, 63–66, 68

Nasal cavities, 21, 89
Nasal sinuses, 21
Nasal tone, 36
Natural method of singing, 90
Negus, V. E., 36, 39, 56, 90
Nervousness, 4–5, 12
Newman, Ernest, 59
Nodules of attrition, 66–69
Nose, diseases of, 80

'Open throat', 89
Over-use of voice, 7

Pachydermia of larynx, 74
Paget, R. A. S., 35, 36
Pain relievers, 78
Penicillin, 78, 91
Personal relationships, 8
Personality, 46, 87
Pharynx, 26, 35, 38
  anatomy, 20
  constriction, 37
  examination, 41
  resonating cavities, 18–20
  role of, 16
Phonasthenia, 63–66
Pitch, 16, 26

Pitch (*contd.*)
  accuracy of, 44
  compass and tessitura, 44
  determination of, 17
  factors affecting, 25
  fundamental, 25
  limitations of, 52
Pitch control, 23, 24
Politicians, 13
Polypi, 80
Post-nasal drip, 92
Pressman, J. J., 66
Prestige, 87
Previews, 83
Producers, advice for, 82
Psychological factors, 1, 7–9, 11, 75, 87
Puberty, 55, 56
Purgatives, 81

Quality (timbre), 16, 25, 59, 89
  assessment, 45
  factors affecting, 25

Reassurance, 9
Recordings, 83
Reed instrument, vocal mechanism as, 15, 16
Registers, 28, 29, 54, 89
Rehearsals, 83
Resonance, 18, 34, 51, 89
  double, 35
  requirements, 35–36
Resonating cavities, 18, 20, 21
Resonator action, 26
Resonator tuning, 28
Resonators, 16
  requirements of, 38
  structure and function of, 34
Respiratory tract, 21
Rest, indications for, 7, 56, 57, 65, 71, 72, 78, 90
Rheumatism, 69
Rhythm, 46
Robson, Frederick, 5
Russell, G. O., 34

Salesmen, 13

Schatz, H. A., 42
School-teachers, 12
Seashore, C. E., 42
Semon, F., 43
Sensitivity, 4
Shakespeare, W., 49
Sicca syndrome, 73
Singers, characteristics of, 1
Sinuses, 80
Smoking, 59, 60–71, 73
Sore throat, 77
  'clergyman's', 12, 75
Sound waves, 30, 89
Steroids, 81
Stimulants, 92
Style, 46
Sundberg, J., 37

Tauber, Diana, 43
Terry, Ellen, 5
Tessitura. *See* Vocal range
Tetrazzini, L., 5, 43, 54
Throat
  damage to, 59, 61
  dry, 11, 71, 74, 76
  health of, 91
  inflammations, 61
  size requirements, 90
  uncomfortable sensations, 74
'Throaty tone', 36
Thyroid dysfunction, 81
Timbre (quality), 16, 25, 59, 89
  assessment, 45
  factors affecting, 25
Tobacco. *See* Smoking
Tone colour, 58
Tone quality. *See* Quality
Tonoscope, 44
Tonsillitis, 77
Tonsils, removal of, 79
Trachea, 21, 36
Traditions, 86–92
Tranquillity, 4
Treatment, 62
Tuberculosis of larynx, 80
Tumours, 80
Tyndall, J., 34

Understudy rehearsals, 84
Upper respiratory inflammation, 7,
  75–79

Vaccines, 76
Vibration of vocal cords, 15–17, 22,
  41
Vibrato variation, 27, 37
Virus infections, 76–77
Vitamins, 76, 80
Vocal cords, 15, 26
  anatomy, 17, 18
  damage to, 26
  defects of, 88
  diagrammatic representation of,
    20
  lubrication. *See* Lubrication
  medicaments intended to improve
    condition of, 91–92
  nodules of attrition, 66–69
  requirements for fine singing, 33
  role of, 16
  thickening and roughening, 70
  vibrations of, 15–17, 22, 41
Vocal dysfunction, 6, 8, 13
Vocal exercising, 56
Vocal mechanism, 14–31
  as reed instrument, 15, 16
  damage risk, 6
Vocal range
  differences in, 29
  problems of, 52–56
Vocal tone, 10
Voice, care and use of, in health,
  48–60
Voice assessment, 40
Voice break-down, prevention and
  treatment, 61–81
Voice 'breaking', 55, 56
Vowel sounds, 16, 26, 35, 37

Walshe, W. H., 42
Wood, Alex, 34, 36
Wyke, B. 26
Wyke, B. D. 27